MW01056905

Old English Medical Remedies

For Jan

Old English Medical Remedies

Mandrake, Wormwood and Raven's Eye

Sinéad Spearing

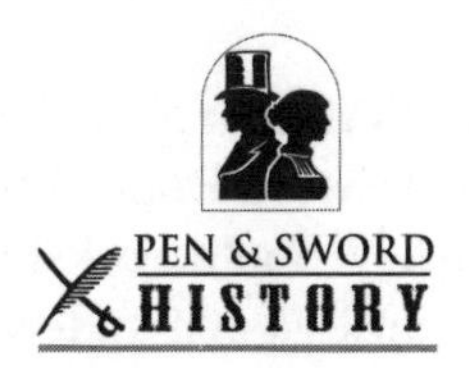

First published in Great Britain in 2018 by
PEN AND SWORD HISTORY
an imprint of
Pen and Sword Books Ltd
47 Church Street
Barnsley
South Yorkshire S70 2AS

ISBN 978 1 52671 170 0

A CIP record for this book is available from the British Library

Printed and bound in England
by TJ International Ltd, Padstow, Cornwall

Typeset in Times New Roman by
CHIC GRAPHICS

Pen & Sword Books Ltd incorporates the imprints of Pen & Sword
Archaeology, Atlas, Aviation, Battleground, Discovery,
Family History, History, Maritime, Military, Naval, Politics, Railways,
Select, Social History, Transport, True Crime, Claymore Press,
Frontline Books, Leo Cooper, Praetorian Press, Remember When,
Seaforth Publishing and Wharncliffe.

For a complete list of Pen and Sword titles please contact
Pen and Sword Books Limited
47 Church Street, Barnsley, South Yorkshire, S70 2AS, England
E-mail: enquiries@pen-and-sword.co.uk
Website: www.pen-and-sword.co.uk

Contents

Acknowledgements

I would like to express my deep gratitude to my husband Jeremy Spearing. Not only did he suggest the subtitle for this book but also he boosted my confidence and supported me in every moment, which culminated in reading the entire manuscript without complaint and giving positive, encouraging feedback. A special word of gratitude is due to my friend, poet and writer Siân Thomas, who has read and commented on a number of chapters and also picked up my confidence when it waned, often. I am particularly grateful to Consultant Psychiatrist Dr Nik Gkampranis whose expertise not only adds to my work but also brings an important level of professional reasoning and support to the murky subject of Old Hags. Thank you for your kindness and time.

Of the many other people who were instrumental in their contribution, my brother, Dr Tom Swan, deserves my thanks for his academic support and like-minded conversations, similarly physiotherapist Jonathan Hockey, for encouraging me to think about these remedies from a more scientific point of view whilst curing my frozen shoulder. Thank you.

My thanks also go to herbalist Susan Tosoni, who kindly offered her professional opinion on the herbal oddity of the nightwalker charm. The Museum of Witchcraft and Magic at Boscastle has also been extremely kind in supplying an image of one its notorious little poppets.

This book would never have been published, however, were it not for the wonderful team at Pen and Sword Books, particularly Lauren Burton, Carol Trow and Jon Wilkinson, who helped bring these pages to life, and Jonathan Wright for his generous feedback and for his confidence in my work. A mention must go to another Pen and Sword author, Willow Winsham, whose excellent book *Accused*, inspired me to send in my own proposal.

ACKNOWLEDGEMENTS

A number of others who provided help or inspiration are Professor Brian Bates, Stephen Pollington and the AncientBiotics group at Nottingham University, particularly microbiologist Freya Harrison and Dr Christina Lee.

* * *

The author does not recommend using or recreating any of the remedies within this book. Many of the cures use ingredients known and proven to be poisonous and deadly. They are explored here for literary and cultural purposes only. Please consult a qualified medical practitioner if you are suffering from or experiencing any medical or psychological complaint, symptoms or concerns.

Introduction

Hidden deep within the British Library is a manuscript of ancient healing remedies, catalogued inconspicuously as Royal 12, D xvii. Penned in the now obsolete language of ninth century Old English, it is a collection of books and manuscripts, the contents of which are even more ancient, being a repository for the herbal therapies, charms and exorcisms of Dark Ages Britain. Intended for use in healing, these enigmatic works have received little attention outside of academe. For those interested in arcane history, however, the text commonly known as Bald's *Leechbook III* reveals within its 109 pages ancient and compelling evidence of folk customs about medicine, magic and a shadow world of demons, elves and other supernatural creatures.

These manuscripts are also a valuable source of information about the common folk of Dark Ages Britain. The Dark Ages have become a time lost to humanity and in our modern world, where information and knowledge are prized, this mysterious period of history which spans from about 400 to 900 AD is in many ways a puzzle still to be solved. Following the fall of the Roman Empire and the gradual withdrawal of its legions, there was an influx of barbarians into Northern Europe who swept away the fledging Christian Church and introduced new pagan beliefs whilst enabling the revival of existing traditions.

Few primary sources of information survive from this forgotten era and so we are fortunate in England to be one of a small number of countries in Northern Europe to have magico-healing texts dating back over a thousand years. Although some of the manuscripts such as *The Old English Herbarium* (attributed to Apuleius Platonicus) are, in part, copies of classical works, Bald's *Leechbook III* and the *Lacnunga*, are almost purely British and consist of herbal remedies and healing charms for all manner of ailments. There are the usual culprits such as dysentery, cysts, problems with childbirth and haemorrhoids, but also included are less familiar ailments such as remedies for evil elves, nightwalkers, the moon mad and those who have sex with the devil.

Within the pages of Bald's book is the phrase, 'Bald owns this book which he ordered Cild to compile' (*Bald habet hund librum Cild quem conscribere iussit,)* which states with admirable brevity the names of the men who respectively commissioned and wrote the *Leechbook*. Little more is known of either of them except that the manuscript was most probably penned in Winchester's great monastic settlement, Winchester being the capital of Anglo-Saxon Wessex. The *Leechbook* may have been a first attempt to develop a medical manual for Anglo-Saxon doctors, and the monasteries would have considered such knowledge extremely valuable.

Bald's *Leechbook*, as it survives today is a copy of an earlier manuscript from the sixth century which was compiled from earlier sources. It should be noted that the word leech does not mean the blood-sucking creature we are familiar with. In Old English 'leech' meant to heal, so leechbooks were considered by their compilers to be healing texts. *Lacnunga*, meaning 'remedies', is a slightly later work, thought to have originated in Northumbria although new evidence suggests Winchester also.

The lack of classical imports and the spattering of Old Irish in Bald's *Leechbook III* suggest this text was sourced from earlier oral folk traditions, from the first Anglo-Saxon settlers who still retained contact and shared healing traditions with the Romano-Britons. As the scholar Malcolm Cameron agrees:

> '*Leechbook iii* reflects most closely the medical practice of the Anglo-Saxons while they were still relatively free of Mediterranean influences,'
>
> (Cameron, *Anglo-Saxon Medicine*, 1993)

More than this, however, is evidence of far older spiritual traditions, pre-dating the religious dichotomy of Christian/pagan so often considered to be the only relevant aspect of these manuscripts. Pagan religions are marked by a plurality of gods, yet within *Leechbook III* and the *Lacnunga* we can literally look back into the distant past, before even this pagan plurality emerged.

Beneath the Christian post-structures, we find the occasional reference to heathen gods such as Odin, but more prominent are the conceptual embodiments of nature that represent a time before even the pagan gods existed. Within the supernatural world populated by ogres, elves, witches, hags and nightwalkers, we find expressed the existence of emerging identities rather than the defined representations of gods and goddesses which formed into what we today understand as pagan beliefs. These emerging identities demonstrate an earlier experience of religious impulse, where forces of nature such as the wind, storms, disease and death are found characterised within the domains of supernatural creatures such as goblins and dark-elves.

Positive natural forces such as light and the sun were also embodied within creatures such as light elves and certain magical plants and animals. This force of light for example, then evolved though the pagan era into identities such as the goddess Eastre/Eostre with her symbols of birth such as eggs, rabbits and hares. Eastre became the inspiration for the Christian festival of Easter, so all three, the force of nature, the pagan representation and the contemporary Christian festival retain the element of light, rebirth and renewal through creation. They are simply conceived and celebrated in differing ways, evolving from ancient primal experience into divine concept.

In early Christian Europe, magic such as we find within these manuscripts fitted comfortably within society. Saints, monks and pagan healers all used these remedies, charms and further magical principles to heal their people during a time when distinctions between the natural and supernatural were not as differentiated as they are today. *Leechbook III* and *Lacnunga* are therefore a unique window into our ancestral past. They stand witness to a time when magic and medicine were interrelated and the new monotheistic religion had not yet become overtly hostile to its host.

A further theme within this book is that of the emergent psychology of the unknown. The role of bacteria, viruses and the importance of hygiene were not understood by the Anglo-Saxons and as will become clear, their response to this unknown threat to health becomes mythologised within a supernatural cosmology. Central to their perspective was the belief that healing was a combined biological and psychological process. Today, modern medicine largely differentiates between the mind and body, separating subjective experience from objective medical intervention. These distinctions arose within pre-modern physics when the material world became ostracised and superior to the immaterial, forcing the human mind and its subjectivity to be separated as psychology with little causal or aetiological connection to physicality. Interestingly, contemporary physics seems to be returning to an interconnected worldview, where psychology and physicality are again interdependent so mind is no longer separated from matter. Our ancestors may not have voiced their beliefs using scientific language, yet it is plain from the texts that knowledge of this interdependence of states existed for them, albeit intuitively, indicating a degree of ontological sophistication.

Archaeological evidence discovered at Bronze Age sites such as the Peterborough Pompeii hint at a sophistication not usually associated with the British Bronze Age and is forcing a re-evaluation of the past. Further discoveries, including the Anglo-Saxon town found near Little Carlton in 2016, also challenge previously held academic views that pre-modern England was a barbaric place. I suggest that the Anglo-Saxon medical texts should join this re-evaluation, although the reluctance is understandable. How are we to attend to remedies that heal the 'moon mad' and those 'who have intercourse with the devil'? How are such odd beliefs to find relevance and place within a modern narrative?

Today many Christians and clergy view these texts as witchcraft, with modern pagans often viewing them as monastic Christian works. Ciaran Arthur argues for example that they demonstrate the early Christian Church attempting to rewrite its authority over the traditions of the people, whilst other researchers suggest these texts demonstrate a continuation of pagan beliefs in a Christian world. Consequently, the religious context of these works has over-shadowed their medical relevance for decades. This lens of religious tension between Christian and pagan influences has caused, and continues to cause these texts to be largely dismissed by researchers as having nothing more to offer.

Although this dualistic religious interpretation is warranted, despite current academic fashion which eschews it in favour of a wider methodology, it is only by interrogating the apparent religious dualism that the underlying syncretic nature of the time can be fully appreciated, freeing the ancient material to speak as witness to a liminal, transitional religious time, 'when both Christianity and Anglo-Saxon paganism existed dynamically side-by-side, and in hybridised forms,' (Saunders, 2013).

Yet a difficulty remains. The cures contained within Bald's Leechbook III and Lacnunga are simply not remedies as we would understand them today and so the process of exploring them to provide a useful interpretation forms much of the aim of this book, and revealing the underlying cosmological belief system and practical methodological applications for healing follow from this interpretative process. For example, our ancestors held a cosmological view quite different from our own. They believed in the living reality of the Otherworld, a realm of powerful supernatural forces recognised as tangible beings responsible for illness and disease. It is necessary to appreciate the reality this metaphysical cosmology assumed for our ancestors, in order to explore the more unusual elements of healing and to make informed suppositions regarding them.

The Otherworld was composed of many realms, some close to us and others far removed. Our own physical world was in the middle, known therefore as middle earth (or *middengeard* in Old English). Professor Brian Bates has argued this cosmological view to be essentially shamanic, sharing elements from primitive pagan cultures throughout the world. His thesis draws the Anglo-Saxon medical practitioner into a wider cultural family of magic workers. Bates uses the term shaman to describe Anglo-Saxon healers and sometimes the word *wicce*, a word that evolved in the Middle Ages to mean witch. Both terms have become corrupted and dispersed, however, and the use of the word witch has particularly accumulated many loaded and negative implications. I prefer to use the term folk-healer in this book when referring to the original practitioners of these Old English remedies.

Further to the unusual cosmological nature of belief structures in Anglo-Saxon Britain are the more uncommon elements of the Old English folk-healing tradition such as elves, ritual and superstitions. These beliefs, such as the actions of elves to cause disease, so often viewed as pagan nonsense may in contrast be the very psychological tools that elevated ancient healing to a mental as well as a physical process, presenting the Old English folk-healing tradition as a holistic approach to healthcare that saw a role for the mind within healing, in contrast to the allopathic, classical principles of our modern medicine.

So what we term 'magic' by today's standards, might be viewed as a sophisticated homeopathic understanding of the nature of disease and infection, and further, this pre-cedes the New Thought movements of the nineteenth century that continue today. New Thought refers to the spiritual and religious groups who view illness as having non-physical cause and at the extreme, to be unreal. Although not going as far as to state the unreality of disease, our ancestors did view many causes of illness as non-physical.

Magical principles then formed our ancestor's methods of healing, with magic acting as the dynamic agent that caused change to occur, collapsing physical and supernatural elements into a unified result. Belief in this powerful action of magic grew from natural observation that sometimes 'like' appears to attract 'like' and consequently, connections between people and objects might be exploited to encourage healing. Recognising and using these sympathetic relationships added an extra layer of application to ancient methods of healthcare. Similarities between mandrake root and the human body, or a raven's healthy eye in comparison to a patients swollen one, could augment the actions of herbal poultices and tonics.

This belief that like attracts, or is in relationship with like, is the basis of modern homeopathy. It is also a principle of entanglement theory in the unusual world of quantum physics.

This healing methodology is then enhanced with ritual, storytelling, exorcism, initiation and psychedelics to produce a healing event which may call upon ancient forces, heathen gods and Christian prayer. Remedies such as the *The Nine Herbs Charm* and *A Sudden Stitch,* both famous among Anglo-Saxon researchers as examples of the strange and mysterious world of Old English medicine demonstrate these healing events in action and also reveal a strong animistic quality to the cures, with herbs assuming powerful identities within a ritualistic landscape. Both remedies are ancient and have undergone much religious evolution as each culture moulded it to better represent its own worldview. Although we may never know their original form, the process of development from pre-historic to modern belief is valuable and delivers an enigmatic result that retains a feeling of something primordial. These cures are excellent examples of ancient medico-magical healing remedies working to affect positive transformation.

Perhaps the most challenging aspect of the Old English folk-healing tradition facing us today, however, is the inclusion not just of elves, but supernatural creatures such as hags, nightwalkers and succubae. It may be surprising to find mention of such things in healing texts written by monks, but these creatures were considered very real by our ancestors, pagan and Christian alike. We might understand them better as psychological unconscious content with the hag, for example, representing our deepest, most primal fears regarding survival and procreation, which have become mythologised as the evil hag. The nightwalker may be a similar expression of unconscious trauma, as it features in a number of remedies with a particularly dark flavour.

Nightwalkers are also mentioned in the poem *Beowulf* and they appear eerily similar to what we would today call vampires, leading me to the reasoned assumption that within these manuscripts we may have evidence of an ancient English vampire tradition. To those familiar with the vampire legends, it may be interesting to learn that vampires feature in the leechbooks at all when Carol Senf states, 'England had no native tradition of vampires' and Konstantinos comments that, 'Great Britain and France do not have any notable, original vampire folklore.' Any stories, myths and literature in England that tell tales of vampires have always been thought to be imports, predominantly from the Renaissance when the first literary romanticisation of vampires began to occur. Summers and Lecouteaux have unearthed a modest history but neither expand their findings, or travel further back than the medieval era.

These formidable researchers and many more like them can easily be forgiven for their conclusions, however, as few of them would ever think or even desire to search through Old English or Irish texts written in language now obsolete. Yet languishing within one certain text is a remedy that aims to protect a person from the unwanted attentions of nightwalkers. Nightwalkers in the context of this ancient cure are categorised along with evil elves and soul sucking succubae and certainly seem indicative of a vampire.

There is no doubt that our ancestors feared nightwalkers and their kind. Archaeologists have unearthed many Anglo-Saxon skeletons buried with stakes through their hearts and their head between their knees, and the inhabitants of one county in England still said prayers for the dead at crossroads well into the twentieth century. An ancient custom from Celtic times advises that one should plant blackberries by the door to ward off nightwalkers. The nightwalker will be so taken by the dark berries that he will be transfixed, unable to stop counting them until dawn.

There is a spiritual pathology evident within these darker remedies, where those suffering from psychological and neurological issues are understood within a mythic framework of elves, nightwalkers and attacks from otherworldly spirits. The illness was not therefore thought to be inherent to the sufferer, but rather, psychological illness was viewed as an aberrant energy coming from outside, and therefore, many of these types of cure are the most ritualistic and include supernatural exorcisms.

Yet who were the practitioners responsible for observing, prescribing and conducting these remedies? What class of physician understood the empirical complexities of behaviours and symptoms that might require an intervention against the advances of a nightwalker, or a herbal concoction including sheep's dung to cure a lesser complaint? Archeological evidence combined with literary and documentary research is beginning to paint a picture of a uniquely female medical and priestly profession in Anglo-Saxon Britain that has disappeared from the historic record. Named 'cunning-women' by archeologists' Tania Dickinson and Audrey Meaney, a phrase describing the very high level of knowledge these women possessed as 'cunning' means 'knowledge' in Old English, these women may be the voices behind Bald's *Leechbook III* and *Lacnunga.* Yet today those voices seem silent.

Although the full journey of the demise of so called 'cunning-women' is a complex one, certain themes surrounding gender, religion and societal power can be discerned. For a class of healing women who also commanded a spiritual influence over local populations to live peaceably with the incoming patriarchal Church of Rome, was not, unfortunately, possible. As doctrine evolved in the early Church and was formulated within a number of documents to become Canon Law, 'Man's superiority was ordained in all matters of life' (Jeanne Achterberg, 1990).

Woman as healer and priestess did not fit within a Christian cosmology. Furthermore, the mystery and sacredness of birth and sexual union became washed over with shame and guilt as Church Fathers sought to interpret scripture to fit a particularly anti-female narrative, that would gradually turn cunning-women into witches and women generally into Satan's vessels. Emblems of femininity such as the womb, became toxic as St Augustine labeled the cause of Original Sin genetic saying that 'the guilt from our origin… was contracted by birth'. Where previously sin had been viewed in more spiritual terms, Augustine collapsed it into duality and brought sin into the very body of Eve (Eve meaning life), causing an infection of evil so that, 'Discord between flesh and spirit becomes our new nature'.

For the Old English folk-healing tradition where spirit and nature were interdependent and complimentary, this dualistic ontology would probably have been alien and baffling. What was good, wholesome and powerful became evil, shaming and evidence of mankind's inherent weakness. The inner conflict this view displays and encourages remains with us today, influencing every aspect of culture and society.

Contextualising these remedies within the cosmological and cultural reality of the time is therefore an important aspect of this book, as it is by doing so that new knowledge may be discerned to inform the present day. For example, in 2015 a number of major newspapers reported that students from Nottingham University had re-created one of the salves from Bald's Leechbook. It includes garlic, onion/leek and the bile of a cow, and much to the surprise of the students, it acted as an antibiotic. Further research found it to be so potent an antibiotic, that it consistently cures the superbug MRSA.

A new area of medical research has now begun called AncientBiotics where remedies such as those within Bald's Leechbook and Lacnunga are being seen with new eyes. This is welcome news for these forgotten texts. This book adds to their work by showing that the ritualistic and supernatural elements are equally important as they reveal a psychologically sophisticated approach to health where allopathic responses alone were not considered efficacious.

It is important to note that not once within these manuscripts or others similar to them, such as the herbal of St Augustine, do we find any mention of the words magic, spell or charm. The Anglo-Saxons had many words for magic, sorcery, spells and charms, yet there is no mention of them here unless the remedy itself is a cure against one. It is we who have cast these remedies as magical charms.

Unfortunately, to describe these remedies as charms encourages the misunderstanding that these prescriptions are simply pagan magic, yet to judge and evaluate ancestral beliefs and customs based upon current notions of what constitutes magic or even paganism, is disingenuous. For example, to bind the herb plantain around the head of a migraine sufferer using red thread, or to face west whilst tracing three circles around the herb selago was not erroneous magic to our ancestors, it was an important aspect of their medical practice.

Regardless of how dismissive we may be of such supernatural adherences today, it is useful to look beyond current beliefs and attempt, as far as possible, to understand these medical practices as they were intended within the time and culture of the era. As Clay Routledge wrote in *Psychology Today* (31/10/15), 'Supernatural forces contribute to the feeling that life is meaningful,' and in the same edition:

> 'Think you don't believe in magic? Think again. Our brains are designed to pick up on patterns: Making connections helped our ancestors survive. You're not crazy if you're fond of jinxes, lucky charms, premonitions, wish fulfillment, or karma, you're just human.'

We all engage in rituals on a daily basis from the habitual routines of getting up and leaving the house in the morning, to athletes' often elaborate good luck rituals before their sporting competitions. Rituals and magically superstitious activities are evolutionary psychological constructs that help us to find meaning and control within the complexity of life. Although the Church can sometimes argue that a problem with such beliefs is that they appeal to human will-power (or even demons) rather than God and are thus evil, this is to perhaps miss the point that almost every activity we engage with today such as taking vitamins, studying for exams, and even locking the doors at night are also acts of will based upon human knowledge, expectations and observation of our world.

Furthermore, if our ancestors made their rituals focus upon a pagan god this was because, from their perspective, no other was yet present. Pagan gods predate the Christian God, and Christianity grew within the foundations and customs of Roman and European paganism. An impulse towards worship did not emerge spontaneously in the first century; human beings have searched for divinity for thousands of years. We were all pagan or pre-Christian at one time and the texts *Bald's Leechbook III* and *Lacnunga*, although containing what we term magic, ritual and superstition, are Old English medical codices used by Christians, written down by Christians and catalogued within England's greatest monasteries.

Chapter 1

The Embarrassment of Bald

Bald had no notion of the controversy his work would inspire in recent times, and how the third volume of his medical treatise would be reviled by some of his modern church brethren as Satan's work. Today, Bald's medical codex has been predominantly viewed through a lens of religious duality, a contrast further supported by the action of transcription and translation. Yet is this dualistic evaluation fair, or is it a product of biased cultural response?

Bald collected and had Cild write down, a vast number of healing remedies and customs that existed in England during the Dark Ages, creating three volumes in total. Before Bald's endeavour, the source of medical knowledge for the monasteries came exclusively from Arabic and Greco-Roman herbals, Pliny's *Naturalis Historia* (77-79CE) and Galen's *Simplicibus* (2CE) being two of the earliest and most notable. Such works were detailed with healing remedies, illustrations and folklore; however, the remedies of the Classical World were not always replicable, as England had its own native flora.

The third volume of Bald's *Leechbook* indicates a desire in the late Anglo-Saxon period to accumulate healing knowledge from local traditions rather than relying solely upon imported texts. This trend is continued in works such as *Lacnunga* and the books of Saint Hildegard, which also catalogue remedies from local populations of Northern Europe, as the local people had their own unique folk-healing traditions that had never previously been transcribed.

The first volume of Bald's work deals with external illness and his second with internal complaints, creating an organised glossary of medical treatments. The content of these two volumes has much in common with Mediterranean herbals. The third book is markedly different, however, representing remedies that did not conform to the first two volumes' aims and further, presents cures that have a particularly different, supernatural character. The *Lacnunga* text is a similar affair, as it contains remedies which appear particularly obscure and magical to the modern reader.

The differences between Bald's third book and his first two volumes are stark, with Malcom Cameron suggesting in his 1983 paper *Bald's* Leechbook*: its sources and their use in its compilation*, that:

> 'The third book is a collection of medical recipes, of lesser scholarly import, entirely separate from and unrelated to Bald's Leechbook.'

Bald's *Leechbook* was compiled in the ninth to tenth centuries in Winchester, probably in the Benedictine cathedral priory of St Peter, St Paul and St Swithun. It is predominantly written in Old English with some Old Irish and Latin as well as unidentified words. Scholars agree that Bald and Cild are unidentifiable. I suggest, however, that Bald is most likely to be Ælfheah the Bald, first English Bishop of Winchester (934-951). The date and location are perfect and although modern surname research finds the name Bald emerging from a small area of Scotland, the name Ecgbald was in existence in Anglo-Saxon England independently, with bald meaning sharp and strong.

It seems clear that with Ælfheah the Bald, the use of the word Bald is similar to that of a nickname. The use of nicknames was common in Anglo-Saxon England and for Ælfheah the Bald to be shortened to 'Bald' would be characteristic of the time. A previous Bishop of Winchester was named Ecgbald, and Ælfheah may also have assumed part of his name to provide continued legitimacy for his own position. Bald was obviously a powerful individual, as Cild asserts that Bald had ordered him to compile the codex, placing Bald in a position of authority.

Cild is an Anglo-Saxon word meaning child and was commonly used as a nickname to denote the favoured offspring of a noble family.

Such children were often sent for their education to a monastery, many working as scribes in the scriptorium. Cild was likely an important charge with few being able to command authority over him. These noble children were normally charged to the Bishop.

The Diocese of Winchester is one of the oldest in England and covered territory from the South Coast to Southwark in London. Ælfheah the Bald studied in the court of King Athelstan and may have been a relation of St Dunstan, Abbot of Glastonbury who became Archbishop of Canterbury in 960. With such illustrious family ties, he may have wished to make his own, personal mark when becoming Bishop of Winchester and as a champion of Church reform and education, an English codex of healing remedies may well have formed part of his agenda.

The third book of Bald's codex suffers from a number of transcriptional difficulties and linguistic uncertainties. Local oracular Irish, Cornish and pre-Old English dialects are evident within a number of remedies, and there are some words that defy translation even today. For example, the remedy, *Wið þeofentum luben luben niga efið niga efið fel ceid fel ceid, delf fel cumer orcggaei ceufor dard giug farig pidig delou delupih*, has never been adequately translated and seems garbled by scribes uncertain of the words they were using or hearing. The original import and experiential context therefore, have become lost to us. Cameron considers that Old Irish and other probably obsolete dialects were included in the manuscript due to an ancient tradition of travel and migration that saw youngsters seeking shelter and hospitality within foreign lands. So scribes, versed in Old English and Latin, may have been transcribing words and languages they had never before heard from a context of folk customs so alien that all we have today is a shadow of their actual import. Furthermore, the original translator of these works, Reverend T. Oswald Cockayne, believed that a large amount of early English words were simply never written down at all and have become lost.

When studying the texts, this linguistic confusion is increased by the problems of transcription and then translation. Cockayne accomplished the first translations into Modern English in the nineteenth century, his painstaking work culminating in the 1864 publication of *Leechdoms, Wort-cunning and Starcraft of Early England*. A number of scholars, including Anne Van Arsdall, argue that Cockayne's work has resulted in a biased view of Anglo-Saxon texts, rendering them literary curiosities rather than offering anything meaningful to the historic record of medicine, Cockayne being guilty therefore of viewing these works as unsophisticated nonsense:

> 'Cockayne's emphasis on the magical, superstitious, and non-rational elements in … medieval medical works has contributed to a generally negative and close-minded perception of medieval medicine generally.'
>
> (Arsdall, *Medieval Herbal Remedies*, 2010.)

Arsdall's criticism echoes that of many modern researchers who eschew dualistic methodological inquiry into Anglo-Saxon medical manuscripts and argue for a more nuanced response. The dualistic methodology is twofold yet contingent; the lens of religious duality of Christian verses pagan, combined with a dualism of sophistication whereby the classically inspired remedies are seen as intelligent and the Old English remedies are by contrast illogical hokum.

I do not believe, however, that Cockayne identified Anglo-Saxon medicine as distinctly supernatural in contrast to that of Classical Medicine out of hand. His distinction between the two, which has indeed informed modern interpretation, evolved from the material itself. He identified, as did his contemporaries, that there was something qualitatively different between the herbariums and codices based upon or drawn from classical works, and the unique texts of *Leechbook III* and *Lacnunga*. I would suggest therefore that Cockayne was correct to speak of a uniquely Anglo-Saxon or Old English medical tradition, the origins of which are ancient. Cockayne's scathing view of this ancient tradition, however, viewing Old English medicine as barbaric in contrast to the rational learned medicine of the Classical World, was greatly flawed. When speaking of Bald's endeavour, Cockayne even goes so far as to say, 'Bald … may have got some good out of it, he may have learned to think, have begun to discriminate …'

It is not coincidental that the Anglo-Saxon compilers of these two texts chose to document them separately from the classically inspired volumes. They identified, even then, that these particular remedies were something different and did not fit within familiar herbal codices. Further, the medical authorities found in Bald's *Leechbook* are not the great figures of the Mediterranean such as Hippocrates; we find instead mention of Dun and Oxa, both described as being teachers of medicine, yet these names are Old English. It seems there was indeed an English native tradition of medicine and healing that has survived within the two texts, *Leechbook III* and *Lacnunga*. This is not to say that the Anglo-Saxons did not also draw on Classical Medicine, especially in the medieval period.

For such a distinction between English and Mediterranean practices to be identified by researchers and translators is not therefore an injustice to the study of Anglo-Saxon medicine that renders it nothing more than a curiosity but rather, it is a clue that reveals a unique Old English folk-healing tradition:

> 'Although English vernacular medicine of the late ninth to twelfth centuries draws heavily upon the classical and sub-classical tradition, classical authorities are almost never cited. In fact, citations of any kind are very rare, and the majority of authorities cited in texts compiled before the Norman Conquest are themselves English. Only in the twelfth century are Galen and Hippocrates mentioned for the first time. This suggests a rather self-sufficient medical community in England, with limited historical awareness or contact with wider developments.'
>
> (Debby Banham, *Dun, Oxa and Pliny the Great Physician*, 2011.)

Edward Pettit, writing in 2001 agrees with Banham that book three is, 'now usually regarded as a separate work'. Yet this has always been true as Cockayne, the first to discover these manuscripts, felt the same, as did the compilers, and when considering the three volumes of Bald's *Leechbook*, Sir Henry Wellcome, writing in 1912, said of *Leechbook III,* 'what is termed the third part of this work evidently does not belong to it'.

Cockayne's transcription and translation have fuelled the argument against dualistic research methods, yet as has been suggested here, he was simply drawing on the already distinctive properties of the material he was handling. His personal opinion regarding sophistication was adjunct to this process and it is helpful to now turn to his endeavour.

Cockayne was a Cambridge-educated ordained priest, yet his life was one of disappointment as his scholarly achievements were never recognised and after serving as a teacher at a London boys school for twenty-seven years, he was dismissed without further pay or pension due to teaching inappropriate material, such as the subject of Mary's virginity, to his students. He committed suicide just a few years later. Cockayne's achievement is undervalued today, as what he accomplished with his transcription and translation paved the way for future research.

Transcribing the Old English texts is an arduous task and many authors, even notable academics have preferred to use the transcriptions of others rather than study the original documents. This is understandable when you see the documents. Unfortunately, this method does at times result in inaccuracies, some of which have gone unnoticed to the point that fictions are at times presented as facts. For example, in *Lacnunga* there is a remedy to ward off attacks from dwarves, and here is the second part of the charm in Old English followed by Modern English:

'Her com ingangan, in spiderwiht hæfde him his haman on handa cwæð þæt þu his hæncgest wære lege þe his teage on sweoran, ongunnan him of þæm lande liþan, sona swa hey of þæm lande coman þa ongunnon him þæt þa colian, þa com ingangan deores sweostar, þa geændode heo, ond aðas swor ðæt

> *næfrte þis ðæm adlegan derian ne moste, ne þæm þe þis galdor begytan mihte oððe þe þis galdor ongalan cuþe.'*
>
> 'In came a noble spiderwiht with his mantle in his hand, proclaiming that you [the dwarf] were his stallion, he put his cord around your neck and he set forth to travel the land, loudly he began to circle the lands, he cast off a garment so the limbs grew cold, then entered his dear sister, and she had brought this about, and she swore an oath that this should never trouble us, nor those that obtain the power of this charm or those that recite this charm through knowledge.'

In the original document, the Old English script is difficult to decipher. The letters *p, s, f* and *w* are all very similar and there is scarce punctuation or use of capitalisation, along with scribal errors and parts that are difficult to read because of the age of the document. Also, certain letters and words used can be ambiguous with researchers arguing and disagreeing on the word before any translation has even been attempted. *Spiderwiht* (the fifth word of the remedy above) is a good example. Grattan and Singer, translating some of the remedies in 1952, transcribed it from the original as *inwriðen with*. Yet in the original document one can see that the word contains an odd-looking string of letters, a number of which all look like p. It is by analysing the surrounding letters that one can tell Grattan's transcription is wrong. Grattan has also made an error reading the Old English letter ð as *d*. This is a pivotal mistake that obscured the real word from him and caused his further errors regarding the use of *p* when it is a *w*.

The whole remedy relies, however, on the accurate transcription of the word *spiderwiht*. A *spiderwiht* is a supernatural creature that battles the dwarf and cures the illness. If we believe Grattan's translation of *inwriðen with*, then we would be talking about a sort of swaddling garment. Or Jason Fisher, who argues the word to be a scribe's error and that perhaps the word was supposed to be *spiwða,* which means to vomit. This is where context is important and the supernatural element of Old English healing needs to be understood. Neither vomit nor a swaddling garment fit the wider context of the cure. *Spiderwiht* it is.

The first words of the remedy are often confused too. Cockayne made a transcription mistake rendering *Wið dweorh* (Against a dwarf) as *Wið weorh*. Yet many researchers talk today of there being an error in the manuscript. There is no error in the manuscript; the error was Cockayne's. This all goes to demonstrate how important it is to go back to the original source and check for accuracy; this is why, where I analyse a remedy at some depth, I have wherever possible (although not exclusively) referred back to the original documents.

Grattan and Singer made a number of ambiguous transcriptions in the remedy against a dwarf, a further one being *eores sweostar* which can be seen in the original document to be *deores sweostar* (dear sister). Grattan believed that *eores* referred to the pagan earth goddess Eastre or Erce, which is an interesting speculation. Eastre's festival with her symbols of the hare, rabbit and egg continue to be celebrated today in churches and schools across England as part of the Easter devotions. Yet the word is obviously *deores*, and Grattan it seems may have tried too hard to make the text fit a certain pagan point of view.

Next comes interpretation. We can see that the spider is not to be feared, and the words *her* and *hæfde* indicate nobility and status, so we have a respected creature here. The dwarf in the first page of the charm is symbolic of the illness afflicting the victim and the spider is brought in to bind (prevent) the dwarf from doing harm, and so the spider becomes the dominant party controlling the disease. The spider rides the dwarf out into the land where it becomes cooler, sympathetically symbolic of the fever leaving. While the spider is dealing with the fever, its sister comes into the scene to complete the rest of the remedy declaring that no one else will be troubled by the dwarf so long as they understand and can recite this healing cure. The amulet placed around the neck may indicate that a real spider was hung around the neck of the patient, a common Anglo-Saxon practice. The use of the word *galdor* indicates this remedy is to be sung or chanted bringing in a ritualistic element.

In *Lacnunga* we find clues as to the mode of collection of these curious remedies. Where most herbariums and medical codices were copies of classical works, one remedy in *Lacnunga* contains the words 'This is my remedy' and continues in a performative voice. Other remedies specific to *Lacnunga* and *Leechbook III* also use the first person, indicating that, unlike many medieval herbals, these English ones were being collected and dictated from the healers themselves. Medieval herbals are predominantly male oriented manuscripts with their authors using the word man rather than person or woman. Yet in these English texts, when we encounter the performative voice, it is often female, indicating that these Old English healers were perhaps, women.

In pre-Christian society, women often held positions of religious, medical and spiritual power due to the belief that certain women had inherent supernatural abilities. This apparently supernatural element to femininity reflects a deeper narrative and belief in the nature of women that once existed. Women were sometimes viewed as liminal, otherworldly, endowed with abilities of intuition, divination, magic and healing. Although the Roman Church as a patriarchal institution became strong within Anglo-Saxon England, within its esoteric beliefs we still find a strong feminine aspect present, with Pope Benedict XVI having stated for example:

> 'It is necessary to go back to Mary if we want to return to that truth about Jesus Christ, truth about the Church and truth about man.'

It is perhaps surprising, given the status of women in the Roman Church generally, that remnants of an ancient belief in a uniquely female power remain within Christianity. The Old Testament contains many references to a variety of powerful female identities such as Ashara. The New Testament retains this knowledge also, with women being the witnesses to Christ's greatest moments of transformation, his conception, crucifixion, the vigil at the tomb and his resurrection. There appears therefore, to be an ancient instinct towards a feminine understanding of spiritual transformation that contained within its auspices a healing ability.

Bald commissioned the collection of these enigmatic English remedies at a pivotal time when the people of Britain were moving from pagan to Christian, and the supernatural context of illness remained an important aspect of healing. Contrary to later attitudes regarding the use of magic within healthcare, the Old English folk-healing tradition was situated in a culture where ritual, magic and the supernatural were not the simplistic beliefs of naïve folk, they were a sophisticated aetiological landscape that brought meaning and control into a hostile world of pain and suffering. Bald need not be embarrassed at all.

Chapter 2

Where Strange Creatures Lurk

Central to the healing practices and religious lives of our ancestors was a mysterious realm that has been termed the Otherworld, a supernatural dimension inhabited by mythic creatures such as elves, dwarves, hags and nightwalkers. It was also home to the spirits of the dead. This may seem bizarre to us today, yet in a time before the aetiology of illnesses were known, our ancestors required a causal psychological framework in which to narrate and understand the reasons for disease. If causality could be fathomed, then healers and their patients could engage in a therapeutic intervention that was meaningful to them and the Otherworld provided this framework of reference. The Otherworld was therefore considered as real as the physical world, even though it contained:

> '... gods, demons, the dead, fabulous beings, celestial happiness, inhuman tortures, unknown spirits, and modes of life and, on the whole, everything that is not of This World.'
>
> (Jens Peter Schjodt, *Initiation between two worlds,* 2008.)

For the folk-healers of Anglo-Saxon Britain, the Otherworld thus offered a way of understanding and dealing with uncontrollable events such as illness. It was otherworldly creatures that caused disease and made harvests fail, therefore if these creatures could be banished back to their own world, then people had a way of coping with occurrences that seemed random. It is this process of coping which used intention, ritual, herbs and invocations that our ancestors viewed as magic.

Rituals served as structural support for a folk-healer's journeys and communications with beings and entities from the Otherworld. Ceremonies would aid a subtle shift in emotion and consciousness whilst framing the intent of the healing being performed, enabling both worlds to converge on the desired outcome. Yet would this type of focused intention really have any effect on a material level?

Contemporary research has offered some possible support for the belief that intention of thought causes alterations in the physical world. For example, Dr Glen Rein, a cellular biologist working at the HeartMath Research Centre in California tested the effects of human mental and emotional intention upon strands of human DNA. Using three groups, he asked one to hold a vial of donor DNA whilst maintaining a heightened state of emotional positivity. A second group were to hold the mental intention to unwind the strand of DNA and the third group was to do both. Dr Rein found statistically significant differences between the first two groups and the third concluding that a heightened emotional state combined with focused intention could produce material change, in this case, the alteration of DNA.

Although more research is obviously required, it may be that science is beginning to reveal what folk-healers might have intuited, that it is possible under certain circumstances to cause changes to occur in accordance with intention if we adopt a particular frame of mind. Therefore, it may be plausible that ceremonies and rituals enabled folk-healers to attain the emotional high and focused intent that research suggests might be harnessed to produce desired outcomes. We commonly use the term 'magic' to describe such seemingly supernatural processes, although increasingly it reminds us of known physics.

Folk-healers would not have experienced this as a scientific process; for them it seems to have been a personal and relational interaction with supernatural creatures. Our ancestors would make offerings to otherworldly beings and gods to encourage their participation before performing ritualistic processes to ensure the required changes in the physical reality would indeed occur. A blend of invocation and symbolic intention was commonly employed and combined with a powerful use of imagination directed towards the intended goal. Symbols were particularly important as they functioned as intermediate modes of communication between the worlds. As the psychoanalyst, Carl Jung, who developed extensive theories of the unconscious mind states:

> 'The place or the medium of realisation is neither mind nor matter, but that intermediate realm of subtle reality which can be adequately only expressed by the symbol. The symbol is neither abstract nor concrete, neither rational nor irrational, neither real nor unreal. It is always both.'
>
> (C.G Jung, *Psychology and Alchemy*, 1944.)

Believing as they did in the immediacy and intimacy of the Otherworld, Old English folk-healers lived a life where everything was imbued with meaning. For example, the flight patterns of certain birds may be portentous symbols of a good harvest, or the appearance of a large crow could tell of ill fortune ahead. Reality was formed of a web of interdependent relationships where nothing occurred without significance. This web was known by the Old English word *wyrd* (destiny) and it was believed that three sisters, the Norns, wove this web of human fate. In Old Norse, *wyrd* translates as *urðr,* which is also one of the names of the sisters. *Wyrd* and *urðr* are feminine nouns and we shall return to this feminine principle of fate later.

The French mystical philosopher Henry Corbin (1903-78) was particularly influential in igniting interest in the Otherworld. Corbin's work centred upon the mysticism of the East, with his main findings focused on the commonality of the Otherworld. The Otherworld was not a unique concept to Anglo-Saxon England but existed also for the healers of Siberia, the Aborigines of Australia, the ancient Egyptians, the Sufism of the East and further indigenous cultures who described just such a world, including the Christian mystics. It is therefore a common uniting theme and enduring principle within many spiritual systems and beliefs, although it may have been called by different names and conceptualised in disparate ways, depending upon cultural differences through time.

Corbin terms the Otherworld the *Mundus Imaginalis* to indicate the imaginal or symbolic quality of the realm, and he argues that it is our imagination that enables us to relate to the Otherworld and harness its energy. This does not refer to functional or cognitive imagination such as our ability to process images in our mind's-eye, problem-solve or paint pictures. Corbin is suggesting a role of imagination far beyond that which we encounter within normal life.

For Corbin, the Otherworld is a precondition of the material world, meaning that our world would not exist without it. For him, as with some contemporary scientists, the physical world is the actualisation of quantum potential and therefore, the Otherworld encompasses our reality rather than being situated by it. Corbin expressed this in metaphysical terms explaining that although we commonly consider our spirit to be situated within our body or brain, the converse is actually true; the body is encompassed and animated by the spirit. Furthermore, imagination has the ability to connect with and move between the two worlds encompassing our psychological and cognitive functions. We are therefore living in a flowing, energetic life that appears to us in visions, dreams and symbols. Carl Jung believed similarly, writing in a personal letter in 1929 that:

> 'I am indeed convinced that creative imagination is the only primordial phenomenon accessible to us, the real Ground of the psyche, the only immediate reality.'

Jung is certainly attributing a primordial creative quality to the imaginative faculty here and by doing so placing it in a powerful position above both worlds. Using current popular terminology, we could interpret that the imagination in this context thus acts as a language between the two worlds, becoming a liminal code that offers us the ability to liaise between the myriad potentials of the 'quantum' universe. Focusing the imagination in this way could thus collapse specific quantum waves into the particles we desire, thereby manifesting our material world. This is why these thinkers use the descriptions of 'active' and 'alchemical' to describe focused imagination and visualisation. They are pointing towards a very specific process of material creation. Whether the deeper intricacies of quantum mechanics adequately support this position is another matter, but they are being used in popular culture nonetheless to conceptualise metaphysical processes and so become usefully descriptive.

The importance of this flowing imaginative language for our ancestors is demonstrated within an old story so important that it has survived for centuries. There is a curious vignette recorded in the historic account of King Edwin's conversion to Christianity and the killing of the prophesying crow. The Anglo-Saxon Chronicle states that King Edwin, ruler of Northumbria in the early seventh century, converted to Christianity in AD 601 and was baptised by Bishop Paulinus. It was whilst he was on his way to hear the Bishop's instructions to the heathen that the event occurred. The story as follows is recorded in an eighth century manuscript from the Abbey of Whitby:

> 'As the foresaid King and his company were hasting with him to the church, for the catechising of those who were in the bondage not only of heathendom but of unlawful wedlock … then a crow with left-handed omen croaked its harsh note. Whereupon all the throng of courtiers who still were in the public place, hearing the bird, stood in amaze to behold it; as though the new song were not to be truly a canticle to our God in His church, but a false and bootless one.'

The story describes that, whilst on their way to the Bishop's catechism, King Edwin, having forsaken the old gods and relieved his pagan advisors of their posts, came to an abrupt halt due to the sudden appearance of a large black crow which, totally without fear despite the entourage of humans, began to sing with what appears to be great authority. King Edwin may well have been terror-struck by the crow, as he would have recognised this to be an important symbol, yet he was now ignorant of its full meaning without his former advisors. The

Bishop, seeing this as a pagan challenge to God's authority, demanded the bird be shot with an arrow:

> '[He] called to a certain one of his attendants; "Shoot me an arrow speedily at the bird." Which straightway done, he bade both bird and arrow to be kept till, after the catechising,'

The crow was delivered to the King and the still heathen congregation, its death as evidence, so the Bishop presumed, of the superiority and power of the Christian god over the pagan gods who had sent the evil bird. What the Bishop did not know was that, according to Old English beliefs, the bird was intended to die anyway. Crows and ravens were considered to be messengers from the Otherworld. The bird had therefore emerged directly from the Otherworld, sent by spirits to deliver an important message to the King. After the message had been delivered, the bird would have returned to the Otherworld by way of its physical death. Unfortunately for King Edwin, the understanding of the bird's symbolic message remained un-interpreted. The King died soon afterwards, killed by Cadwallon and Penda at Hatfield on the fourteenth of October.

Within the texts, the imaginative faculty is rarely directly referred to and this may be because it was taken for granted. There is, however, one remedy that gives a hint regarding the use of imagination or visualisation within the Old English folk-healing tradition. It's a cure for an adder's bite and here is the remedy in Old and Modern English:

> *'Wið næddran slite genim þas ylcan wyrte þe we ebulum nemdun ond ær þam ðe þu hy forceorfe heald hy on þinre handa ond cweð þriwa nigon siþan, omnes malas bestias canto þæt ys þonne on ure geþeode, besing ond ofercum ealle yfele wilddeor, forceorf hy ðonne mis swyþe cearpon sexe on þry dælas. Ond þa hwile þe þu ðis do þenc be þam men þe þu ðærmid þencst to gelacnienne ond þonne þu þanon wende ne beseoh þu þe na; nim ðonne þa wyrte ond cnuca hy, lege to þam slite, sona he bið hal.'*

> 'For an adder's bite take this same plant which is called ebulum and before you cut it hold it in your hand and say thrice times: "*Omnes malas bestias canto*" which is in our language "I charm and overcome all evil wild beasts" then cut it up with a very sharp knife into three parts, and while you are doing this visualise the person whom you intend to cure therewith, and when you turn from there do not look back at all; then take the plant and pound it, lay it to the bite, he will shortly be well.'

Ebulum is common elder or black elder. In England, it could also refer to dwarf elder. In her 1971 book *A Modern Herbal*, Margaret Grieve, referring to a comment from the physician Michael Ettmueller, says of the plant, 'Elder has been termed the medicine chest of the country people' and 'a whole magazine of physic to rustic practitioners'. Elder has so many medicinal virtues that there seem few complaints it hasn't been used to treat:

> 'If the medicinal properties of its leaves, bark, and berries were fully known, I cannot tell what our country men would ail for which he might not fetch a remedy from every hedge either for sickness or wounds.'
>
> (John Evelyn, *Sylva, or A Discourse of Forest-Trees and the Propagation of Timber in His Majesty's Dominions* , 1664.)

This is praise indeed and when used topically, elder is good for wounds, swelling and inflammation so the site of the bite may well have been relieved. It does not necessarily follow, however, that elder alone would have any significant effect on the venom associated with an adder's bite. Perhaps the focused intention may nonetheless have provided some relief, at the very least creating a placebo effect to promote the bodily fortitude needed to recover.

The ritualistic elements of this remedy demonstrate common motifs from the manuscripts. The number three features regularly in the remedies and is an ancient numeral of power within many spiritual traditions. David Person in *Varieties* (1635) talks of a 'natural triplicity' to life which has become expressed in humanity's understanding of deity. Pagan goddesses such as the Norns and the classical Fates were always depicted as having three aspects understood to be expressions of one unified deity. Christianity retains this notion in its Trinitarian character of God. There is therefore a symbolic wholeness and power to the number three that is used in the charm. Reciting the words 'I charm and overcome all evil wild beasts' three times and cutting the elder into three parts would help ensure the desired intent would find its resolution in healing. The directive to 'not look back' is equally common to the ritualistic devices emerging from the superstition that evil can be transferred through the eyes.

There is an unusual element in the cure for an adder's bite, however, and it is the directive to 'visualise the person whom you intend to cure therewith'. Although extensive anthropological research has found visualisation to form a great part of indigenous tribal practices surrounding healing and religion, this imaginal aspect has rarely been documented outside modern research on indigenous cultures. It has always remained assumed, rather than proven, that our ancestors used it. Here, then, is evidence that our ancestors did indeed use visualisation, imagination and focused intention within their healing practices.

Today, the notion of the Otherworld is receiving increased attention within the fields of academe and psychology and it is interesting to see how such mystery is described in contemporary terms. The scholar James Hillman explains:

> 'Our distinctions are Cartesian: between outer tangible reality and inner states of mind, or between body and a fuzzy conglomerate of mind, psyche and spirit. We have lost the third, middle position which earlier in our tradition, and in others too, was the place of soul: a world of imagination, passion, fantasy, reflection, that is neither physical and material on the one hand, nor spiritual and abstract on the other, yet bound to them both.'
>
> (*The Essential James Hillman: A Blue Fire*, 1990.)

Hillman is expanding upon Jung's notion of the in-between state that he believed manifests within our deep psychology. Jung postulated that it is this third space, uncommon to us today, which is neither interior nor exterior but between the two, a space where imagination may act as a bridge. It might be that Jung is influenced here by the ancient symbolism surrounding the number three, attempting to conceive it in psychological terms.

Another of Jung's contemporaries, the psychoanalyst Marie-Louise von Franz wrote in her 1997 book *The Alchemical Active Imagination* that the Otherworld is:

> 'the plane on which active imagination takes control. With the inner nucleus of consciousness you stay in the middle place … you stay within your active imagination, so to speak, and you have the feeling that this is where your life process goes on.'

Franz specifies her concept of imagination as 'active' and alchemical. This is to bring across the intentional, focused state of visualisation that can, so Franz and Jung theorised, cause changes to occur in our lives, and further, induce a transmutation of consciousness from the lower animal levels to a higher spiritual nature. Imagination, used in this transformational way can then reconnect us with the Otherworld through a shift in consciousness which results in an expansion of awareness. It is not easy to find this middle place and Jung advised that active engagement with the imagination was the best way to explore this transitional state. Jung was naturally suited to this form of inquiry as he came from a spiritual family. His mother was fascinated with the occult and the young Jung experienced many powerful dreams where he conversed with spirit entities as well as his own ancestors. In *Memories, Dreams, Reflections* (1962) he describes one of his imaginal experiences:

> 'I found myself at the edge of a cosmic abyss. It was like a voyage to the moon, or a descent into empty space. First came the image of a crater, and I had the feeling that I was in the land

> of the dead. The atmosphere was that of the other world. Near the steep slope of a rock I caught sight of two figures, an old man with a white beard and a beautiful young girl. I summoned up my courage and approached them as though they were real people, and listened attentively to what they told me.'

Jung's concept of the collective unconscious is very similar to that of the Otherworld, except that Jung mapped out the dominant energies, creatures and impulses of the in-between realm as they appear to us as archetypes, and he characterised the imagination as a magical or alchemical activity capable of causing changes within the physical realm:

> The imaginatio, or the act of imagining, was thus a physical activity that could be fitted into the cycle of material changes that brought these about and was brought about by them in turn'

Categorising impulses and communications from the Otherworld as archetypes enabled a conceptual understanding of the Otherworld. However, although Jung believed the Otherworld to be ontologically real, his development of psychoanalysis resumed a Cartesian flavour, casting it as the working of the unconscious mind, part of our internal psychological processes alone.

Other great thinkers view the imagination as rather more powerful. The Swiss physician and mystic Paracelsus wrote:

> 'It is necessary that you should know what can be accomplished by a strong imagination. It is the principle of all magical action... And this imagination is such that it penetrates and ascends into the superior heaven, and passes from star to star.'
>
> (quoted in Jeffrey Raff, *Jung and the Alchemical Imagination*, 2000.)

Imagination has been argued by these thinkers to be a powerful tool that encompasses both this and the Otherworld, while functioning also as the energy which unites them. It is conceived as a web that connects all things together and it is the foundation upon which everything material is formed.

This active or alchemical imagination is not something we tend to employ in our everyday lives; more familiar to us are the lower activities of the imaginal faculty. We have a cognitive imagination that associates images and solves problems and an egoic form of phantasy that indulges the wants and desires of the bound ego. There is also a creative form of imagination utilised in the arts and finally, we have the alchemical imagination, the transformative function of our higher consciousness.

These levels do not describe distinct categories, as imagination is a constant ability which different human functions utilise in different ways. The ego can employ it to deceive and limit us if we remain unaware of its desires. This is because imagination is morally neutral, neither good nor bad as it exists as Corbin argued *a priori*, before the dualism of corporeal and non-corporeal. Imagination pre-exists our efforts to categorise and evaluate our experiences. It is pre-linguistic. Our use of imagination rarely moves beyond the egoic and creative levels, however, and so it is particularly useful to cultivate self-observation to gain freedom from the egoic level. As the Jungian theorist, Jeffrey Raff, explains:

> 'By seeking the meaning of life events [through the alchemical imagination], the ego escapes from the illusory world of fantasy that only sees concrete reality and appearances. A conflict with a boss, a car accident, a headache.... all of these events may be perceived with the eyes of the imagination. Such a perspective frees one from the sense of being trapped in the situation, and permits one to seek the meaning related to it. Working with meaning opens up possibilities that were hidden before.'

The Otherworld is enjoying a small revival today. New Age gurus such as Eckhart Tolle and Wayne Dyer suggest that there are transitional spaces that they term the 'Now' and the 'Kingdom of God' respectively. These spaces, they explain, are already present. You just need to change your perception by freeing yourself of material bondage and there is a whole new way of being alive. Living in the moment is a strong motif in these New Age approaches, where the consequent is a change of consciousness where both worlds, the outer and inner, merge into a new unified whole, ending duality and revealing the *a priori* truth of our being.

Concepts of the Otherworld continue to evolve, however, with Tolle and Dyer recently giving way to the Secret and the Quantum Field, where quantum mechanics is being used to facilitate notions of ontology that view humanity as being personally responsible for all the good and bad that happens in life. Commonly called the law of attraction, proponents argue that we can bring abundance into our lives by imagining that we already have it. Therefore, the imagination causes manifestation. God is often redundant in this emerging landscape where people are still, in essence, trying to make sense and gain control of a world where chaos and randomness cause insecurity. Even today, many diseases remain incurable and their causes speculative. Elves may offer us little reassurance, but for our Old English ancestors, the creatures lurking in the Otherworld were their only way of bringing some meaningful hope to a difficult situation.

Chapter 3

The Day the Elves Died

When in 1676 Antony Van Leeuwenhoek discovered bacteria, the elves died. The narrative of poisoned arrows being fired from the Elvish Kingdom of Elfame was no longer necessary to explain illness to the mind. Belief in elves had of course, been waning for centuries, yet when at their height, elves were responsible for myriad infections and diseases; because if we as human beings know what the cause of our suffering is, we can formulate a response believable to the mind and hopefully resolve the problem.

Elves and magic rendered the unknown knowable and controllable, consequently providing the mind with a landscape of belief that could aid healing. Uncertainty breeds superstition and we might understand seemingly magical processes today as a placebo effect where the mind, with the correct motivational belief, can affect healing without medical intervention. The Old English folk-healing tradition gave human psychology just as much consideration in healing as the pharmaceutical effect of herbs. For our ancestors, therefore, healing could be said to be a mind-body experience.

Herbs were certainly the foundational element in the majority of leechbook remedies, with some interesting exceptions. Yet even the herbal directives given within the prescriptions are not without their wider psychological context. Collecting herbs was an art in itself, with many remedies indicating particular times, seasons and modes of harvest as well as application. Layered on top of these factors are the rituals and further magical and supernatural principles that combine to formulate a rich and interactive healing experience. Before delving further into the Old English tradition, it is interesting to view our ancestor's healing arts from the perspective of scholars who were, and continue to be, considered as authoritative.

The innate power of herbs fascinated the great first century Roman historian Pliny who wrote an extensive treatise entitled *Natural History* in 77CE. A man obsessed with collecting knowledge that included detailed first hand observations of the indigenous cultures of Northern Europe, Pliny would send his students with the Roman armies to record every detail about the people they encountered and specifically, their religious and magical practices. Within Pliny's observations in Britain he says of the herb vervain:

> 'When it was rubbed on the body all wishes were granted; it dispelled fevers and other maladies; it was an antidote against snakes, and conciliated hearts. Vervain also protected against fear and fantasy, as did holding five leaves from the nettle in the hand.'

Pliny further describes that the herb selago was believed by the British to have:

> 'preserved one from accident, and its smoke when burned healed maladies of the eye, [and also], the diggers do not face the wind, they first trace round the plant three circles with a sword, and then dig up the plant whilst facing west … They then pound root, with rose oil and wine, it cures fluxes and pain in the eyes.'

The circle is a symbol of protection and has been used as such in many religions including Druidism, Buddhism, and early Orthodox Christianity. Tracing three circles with a sword would have amplified the protective intention for a remedy that is designed to 'preserve one from accident'. Pliny also records that indigenous folk-healers of Northern Europe often eschewed using iron tools to dig their herbs and a prescription for a headache from Bald's *Leechbook III* does indeed advise against the use of iron:

> *'Adelf wegbrædan butan isene ær sunnan upgange, bind þa moran ymb þæt heafod mid wræte reade þræde, sona him bið sel.'*
>
> 'Dig waybread without iron and before the sun rises, bind the roots around the head with a red thread, it will soon be better for him.'

Waybread (*wegbrædan*) is the plant we know today as plantain; native to Britain it acts as an anti-inflammatory and is beneficial for all manner of skin conditions and wounds. The recommendation to dig up the plant without the use of iron gives an idea of the age of this particular remedy. Anglo-Saxons and the Britons before them believed iron to be a magical and protective metal, so remedies specifically deriding its use could be due to folk memories of a time when iron was still new and viewed with suspicion.

Even today, new technologies can be held in suspicion. When printing first made books available to everyone, many scorned them as evil temptations from the devil, encouraging idleness. Iron would have been no different. For people accustomed to tending their herbs with wooden implements, iron may have been thought ill-fated or to contaminate in some way. There are numerous directives to avoid iron in the leechbooks, indicating that many of the remedies may pre-date its discovery. To bind a patient's head with a red thread is an act of protection in early Celtic medicine. The thread was used to safeguard people from the actions of malevolent otherworldly spirits, in this case, spirits that may have caused the headache.

A powerful symbol often used in the remedies, especially those with a more pronounced psychological flavour, is the moon. The inclusion of lunar directives in the leechbooks makes it clear our ancestors associated the moon with the mind and the movement of energy, a belief inspired perhaps by the observation of ocean tides and their relationship with the moon's phases. Appeals to the moon were thought to create a sympathetic healing bond with those afflicted with mental illness. One psychological cure prescribes that a bundle of herbs should be collected at the new moon just before dawn. The plants are then to be wrapped in red cloth and tied about the patient's head whilst the moon is waxing. The waxing moon, growing in size and energy, was thought to increase the potency of healing remedies. To banish a spirit or elf thought to be causing a mental illness, however, the cure would be worked during the waning moon, ensuring the creature's hold over the patient would diminish and wane with the lunar cycle.

A further remedy using the moon's phases is recorded in *Lacnunga* and concerns the collection of the herbs periwinkle and mulberry. Periwinkle should be plucked:

> 'when the moon is nine nights old, and eleven nights, and thirteen nights, and thirty nights, and when it is one night old.'

Mulberry should be collected:

> 'when to all men the moon is seventeen nights old, after the meeting of the sun, ere the rising of the moon.'

Twilight, and the moments just before sunrise were auspicious times for the collection of herbs. These marginal spaces between light and dark were believed to be especially potent times of otherworldly connection as these moments represented the transition of knowledge from the unknown to the revealed. Night was also an important time to harvest certain herbs as darkness symbolised things that were hidden from our daily senses. In *Leechbook III* there is a charm for hysteria which uses the marginal time when 'day and night divide':

> *'Leoht drenc wiþ wedenheorte, elehtre, bisceopwyrt, ælfþone, eolone, cropleac, hindhioloþe, ontre, clate, nim þas wyrta þonne dæg ond niht scade, sing ærest on ciricean letania ond credan ond pater noster. Gang mid þy sange to þam wyrtum, ymbga hie þriwa ær þu hie nime ond ga eft to ciricean, gesing xii mæssan ofer þam wyrtum þonne þu hie ofgoten hæbbe.'*

> 'A light drink for a frenzy: lupin, bishopwort, Elfthon, elecampane, cropleek, hindhealth, radish, burdock; take these plants when day and night divide, sing the litany first in church, and the credo, and pater noster, go while singing to the plants, go round them thrice, before you take them and go back to church and sing twelve masses over the plants when you have steeped them.'

The Anglo-Saxon word *wedenheorte* points to more than just a frenzy, it could equally be translated as extreme insanity or violent madness. It is important to consider, however, that what appears to us today as something frenzied and possibly insanely mad, may not have had the same appearance and meaning to our ancestors. We may never know exactly what was meant by frenzy as the categories and observations of what constitute a particular psychiatric issue have changed over time. A document from Victorian England for example, includes within its list of Insane Asylum admissions, the madness of 'novel reading'. Pertinent to evaluating this type of historical data therefore, is the wider social and cultural context, as many Victorian committals for pastimes such as reading novels served an agenda. Husbands with wealthy wives would then have full access to, and control of, their fortune.

We can gain some insight into what *wedenheorte* truly meant for the folk-healer, however, by the actions of herbs and the ritual observations surrounding the 'frenzy'. Bishopswort *(bisceopwyrt)* is a natural preservative and antiseptic. It features in many of the cures and would have provided self-sterilisation for the balms and tonics. It is used in Ayurvedic medicine today. Elfthon (*ælfþone*) is the Anglo-Saxon word for nightshade, a powerful sedative, demonstrating the need within this remedy for an intense soporific action. Elecampane (*eolone)* is commonly used in the remedies as a general tonic. It's known as a safe expectorant and is calming for the stomach; however, it is also a mild stimulant (as is *hindhioloþe)* and may have been used in this context to ensure a balance to the nightshade. I have observed within a number of cures that dangerous ingredients such as nightshade, wormwood and mandrake are often combined with counter-acting agents. This may seem counter-intuitive, yet with the correct quantities it is possible that the folk-healer worked in this way to diminish the worst side effects of the poisonous elements. Cropleek is of the onion family and was thought to draw out illness. Radish has many health benefits and was used as a general tonic, often aiding recovery from illness, as was burdock that added its calmative properties on the nervous system, acting as an antispasmodic.

The ritualistic elements of this remedy have been Christianised from pagan originals. Singing to plants is an ancient custom of empowerment and casting a circle around plants and areas of healing were thought to create protection from negative forces. These magical elements, although often contentious today, made the remedy believable to the patient and healer alike. From their point of view, they were dealing with an attack from otherworldly powers, and herbs alone might help the body, but more was required to thwart the negative spiritual intentions causing the malady. Magic helped to justify the efficacy of the remedy objectively to the mind in a time when subjective experience was dominant.

In the above remedy, we therefore have protective ritualistic elements combined with herbs that deliver strong sedative, restorative and anti-spasmodic affects. These types of pharmaceutical actions may have been beneficial for complaints requiring relaxation of muscles and the nervous system.

Unusually, the next remedy for moon-sickness contains no herbs at all. All researchers have ignored it, probably because it seems bizarre. With no herbal ingredients that can be evaluated within experiments to ascertain their efficacy, we are left, so it seems, with nothing but oddness:

> *'Wiþ þon þe mon sie monaþseoc, nim mereswines fel, wyrc to swipan, swing mid þone man, sona bið sel, amen.'*

> 'For that one be moon-sick, take a dolphin's hide, make it into a scourge, beat the person, he will soon be better.'

Beating a person to health appears counter-intuitive yet there is a long history of using flagellation for medical purposes. Dr. Millingen, writing in 1837 says:

> 'The effect of flagellation, may be easily referred to the powerful sympathy that exists between the nerves of the lower spinal marrow and the other organs.'

Today we understand that the pain response from repeated flogging releases endorphins and adrenaline that can promote a euphoric state and cathartic experience, both of which may calm psychological trauma.

In *The Whip and the Rod* (1948) R. Yelyr states that:

> 'Many readers will find no disagreement with the notion that for the treatment of simulated or imaginary diseases there is nothing more effective than a good whipping.'

Although contemporary readers may find such a statement arguable, Yelyr's book is nonetheless a scholarly treatise on the history of corporal punishment and finds that flagellation has been known as a cure for both physical and imagined illness since pagan times and continued as a favoured remedy through the Christian era. In Canterbury Cathedral, there is a very early thirteenth century window depicting the cure of a mad man. It shows the patient being dragged to the shrine of St Thomas where he is then whipped with rods. The next scene then displays him as cured and thankful.

If a cathartic response is combined with supernatural beliefs, then the effects may be amplified. In medieval times, flagellation was used as a tonic to relieve many complaints from constipation to epilepsy, known as the falling sickness or morbus. The falling sickness was thought to be linked to the changing moon (moon-sickness) and it was this illness that first promoted the modern term lunacy, although we don't associated this word with epilepsy today of course. In later times, as Christianity put many ancient supernatural beliefs under the auspices of the devil, epilepsy became diabolically inspired. W.R. Ward writes regarding epilepsy in his book *Christianity Under the Ancien Regime* (1999), that:

> 'There were sharp limits to what medicine could be expected to accomplish; perhaps exorcism was called for, perhaps it was even a panacea.'

One can imagine that before epilepsy was properly understood, and during a time where subjective experience welcomed supernatural interpretation, that otherworldly sources, be they pagan elves or Christian demons, were the only explanation for such a difficult condition. Moon-sickness was most probably therefore describing what we know today as epilepsy.

The use of dolphin skin in the remedy is particularly unusual, although the animal itself was sacred to the Celts and Anglo-Saxons. In their 2004 paper, *Evidence for an Anglo-Saxon dolphin fishery in the North Sea*, Jeremy Herman and Keith Dobney put forward a fascinating proposition that our ancestors farmed dolphins, most probably for food, so the idea that a scourge could be made from their skin is probable. Researchers from the University of New Mexico and others in Singapore are currently developing synthetic human skin with nanotechnology inspired by the antimicrobial properties of dolphin skin that causes it to heal quickly from wounds. It might be that our ancestors also observed how dolphins healed quickly and this may have contributed to their belief in the healing properties of their skin.

A further folkloric interpretation of the cure emerges from an alternative translation of the word dolphin. The generally accepted translation that I have used here translates *mereswines* as dolphin. The Anglo-Saxons, however, had a specific word for dolphin, *delphin*, and by the time of the writing of the leechbooks, it is likely the accurate word would have been used. It is possible therefore, that *mereswines* means seal.

Our ancestors also held seals in high regard, as they were believed to have magical abilities and could shapeshift into human form. These shapeshifting seals were known as Selkies or Fin-Folk and they inhabited the lands around the North Sea, coming to ancient Britain with the Nordic invaders. It is possible their stories began in relation to the early settlers of Scandinavia (the Saami) who, clothed in sealskin, were thought to be powerful sorcerers. Today, Selkie beliefs survive only in the Orkney Isles and the West of Ireland.

Transition times within the turning of the year are also used in the remedies to bring a further layer of power to their healing practice. In *Lacnunga* there is a remedy for a cyst or tumour upon the neck that utilises the turning from Spring into Summer. Here we can see how the hidden nature of the herbs should be digested directly into the body of the afflicted person at the moment of daylight's revealing:

> *'Se man se ðe biþ on healsoman, nime healswyrt ond wudamerce ond wudsfillan, ond streawbergean wisan, ond eoforþrotan ond garclifan, ond isenheardan butan ælcan isene genumen, ond æðelferðþincwyrt ond cneowholen ond bradbisceopwyrt ond brunwyrt, gesomnige ealle þas wyrta togædere þrim nihtan ær sumor on tun ga, ælcre efenmicel, ond gewyrce to drænce on wyliscan ealaþ, ond þonne on niht þonne sumor on tun gæð on mergen, þonne sceal se man wacyan ealle þa niht, þe ðone drenc drincan wile, ond þonne coccas crawan forman syðe þonne drince he æne, oþre siðe þonne dæg ond niht scade, þridden siðe þonne sunne upga, ond teste hine syþþan.'*

> 'The person who has a neck-tumour: may they take halswort, and wood parsley and wood chervil and strawberry runners and boarthroat and agrimony and ironhard gathered without any iron, and athelfarthingwort and knee-holly and broad bishopwort and brownwort; he may bring all these plants together, the same amount each, for three nights before summer and may go to the farm, and he should make a drink from them in Welsh ale [bragget], and then on the night when summer comes to the farm on the next morning, the person who means to drink the potion must stay awake all the night, and when the cock crows for the

first time he may drink once, a second time when day and night divide, a third time when the sun goes up, and let him rest after.'

Cockayne's contemporaries Singer and Grattan saw this type of remedy as evidence for the ignorance of the Anglo-Saxons. Following Cockayne's belief in the stupidity of folk-remedies, Singer and Grattan suggest that herbs such as halswort (neckwort) were used by reference to their name alone with no consideration regarding healing efficacy. They contend that a homeopathic model of healing (like curing like) was naïve and simple. My research supports the misunderstanding of this point of view. Singer and Grattan's stance relies upon the assumption that the healing attributes afforded neckwort arose from its name. Contrarily, it was the healing attribute that inspired the name. Neckwort has the Latin name *Campanula Trachelium* and other common names include throatwort. It was used for inflammation of the throat as well as wounds relating specifically to the neck.

Directives to face certain directions when collecting herbs or to avoid sunlight altogether also occur in many remedies. The *Lacnunga* recommends that when prescribing sea-holly for healing, 'thou shalt take up this wort with its roots, then beware that no sun shine upon it, lest its beauty and its might be spoiled through the brightness of the sun,' implying that some herbs were considered to be at their most efficacious while still cloaked within the veil of the Otherworld.

A direction for the use of bark within remedies was rather different, with ash and oak to be collected from the side of the tree facing the rising sun. Perhaps this was because the East side was believed to receive the greatest amount of sunlight and was thus strong with life force. It is also possible, however, that our ancestors believed it was the tree's East side where the tree spirit is first witness to the change from dark to light and the knowledge this transient moment reveals.

Portentous days of power feature in Lacnunga. For example, the following remedy is evidence of a belief in days of death:

'Þry dagas syndon on geare þe we egyptiaci hatað, þæt is on ure geþeode plihtlice dagas, on þam is þonne utgangendum þam

> *monþe þe we aprelis hatað se nyhsta monan dæy an, þonne is oþer ingangendum þam monþe þe we augustus hatð se æresta monan dæy, þonne is se þridda se æresta monan dæy æfter utgange þæs monþes decembris. Se þe on þysum þrim dagum his blod gewanige, sy hit man, sy hit nyten, þæs þe we secgan gehyrdan, oþþe gif hwa on þisum dagum acænned bið, yfelum deaðe he his lif gændað, ond se þe on þysum ylcum þrim dagum gose flæaces onbyrigeð, binnan feowortiges daga first he his lif geændað.'*
>
> 'There are three days in the year which we call egyptiaci, that in our language means dangerous days, on which under no circumstances and out of no need is neither man's nor animal's blood to be lessened. That is, at the end of the month we call April, on the next Monday, then the second [day] is at the beginning of the month we call August, the first Monday, the third [day] id then the first Monday after the end of the month of December. Whoever, may lessen his blood on these three days, be it man or animal, according to what we have heard tell, that shortly on the first day or the fourth day, his life shall end, or if his life should go on longer, that he shall not reach the seventh day, or if he drinks some drink on those three days, he shall end his life within fifteen days, if someone shall be born on these days, he shall end his life in an evil death, and whoever eats the flesh of goose on these three days, will, within forty days, end his life.'

In this passage, we see the Old English words for day, which are *dagas* and *dæg*. This becomes more apparent when we learn that the *g* was pronounced as our modern *y*. We also see *deaðe,* which was pronounced as our modern word death.

This is not a remedy or cure, but appears instead to be a warning or instruction based upon 'what we have heard tell', indicating that this is a new belief our ancestors thought it pertinent to adopt. The *egyptiaci* to which they refer, is an ancient superstition from Chaldea (an area of Babylonia during the sixth to ninth centuries BC) that took root in ancient Babylonia in which certain days are considered to be unlucky or dangerous.

The poet Hesiod wrote a treatise entitled *Works and Days*, where he attempted to provide a calendar of these unlucky days for farmers and communities. Proculus and Plotinus also mentioned the *egyptiaci*, and in 398AD, the fourth Christian council of Carthage tried to eradicate the practice as pagan superstition. The Church struggled, as the people were reluctant to give up practices which they believed had served them well for generations. Realising belief in the *egyptiaci* could not be eradicated, the Church decided instead to re-form the belief into a Christian mould. To this end, they changed the most important unlucky days into biblical anniversaries, attributing them as follows: the day of Cain's birth and Abel's death (first Monday in April), the day of the fall of Sodom and Gomorrah (first Monday of August) and the day Judas Iscariot was born (last Monday of December).

Despite the Church's efforts, the *egyptiaci* continued. Writing in the sixteenth century the theologian Thomas Kirchmaier tells us:

> 'And first, betwixt the dayes they make no little difference, for all be not of vertue like, nor like preheminence, but some of them Egyptian are and full of jeopardee, And some againe, beside the rest, both good and luckie bee, like difference of the nights they make, as if the Almightie King, that made them all, not gracious were to them in everything.'

The West Country of England is known to retain many customs regarding portentous days. New Year's Day attracted the greatest superstition, perhaps due to the still existent memory of the old calendar. Moving the New Year was a significant event, and many would have regarded the new date with great suspicion. The beliefs mainly surround the acts of washing and cleaning, acts that had long been symbolic of cleansing negative influences from one's life and environment. Using a besom (broom), it was thought that evil spirits and malicious intentions from others could be literally swept away. The changing of New Year and the suppression of old superstitious days from the Church evolved these old cleansing beliefs into negative ones until it became dangerous to wash clothes, dishes or to clean the house at New Year, as to do so was thought to bring death to the family, as in this account from 1896:

> 'On New Year's Day one of our maids was going to do the family washing, when our West-country girl exclaimed in horror: "Pray don't 'ee wash on New Year's Day. Or you'll wash one of the family away!"'

Superstitions regarding the harvesting of herbs at certain times and on specific days perhaps indicates an ancient instinct for what has today been termed biodynamic agriculture, which refers the growing of plants in harmony with Earth's natural cycles. Although biodynamics is generally believed to have been developed by Rudolf Steiner in the 1920s, these Old English manuscripts may demonstrate an existing heritage of biodynamic knowledge in Northern Europe long before Steiner organised it into the ecological principles known today. His agricultural model recognises that human and plant life respond to lunar and solar cycles and so working within nature's pre-existing ecological system offers the healthiest and most environmentally sustainable farming solutions. For example, biodynamic farmers utilise the influence of the full moon as seeds germinate faster at this time and the water content of soil increases.

Before the elves died, they were the greatest cause of illness for our ancestors and a large number of healing remedies within the leechbooks contain references to their activities. These creatures, unlike the benign elves portrayed in The Lord of the Rings, would fire poisoned spirit arrows into people causing infections and fevers. There were many types of elves such as dark elves (*dökkálfen*), black elves (*svartálfen*) and some light elves (*ljósálfen*). Maladies which had no known cause were often called elf-sickness, and attributed to elves:

'Wið ælfadle nim bisceopwyrt, finul elehtre, ælfþonan nioþowearde, ond gehalgodes cristes, mæles ragu, ond stor, do ælcre hand fulle, bebind ealle þa wyrta on claþe, bedyp on fontwætre gehalgodum þriwa, læt singan ofer iii mæssan, ane omnibus Scis oþre contra tribulatjonem, þriddan pro inwirmis; do þonne gleda an gledfæt ond lege þa wyrta on, gerec þone man mid þam wyrtum ær undern ond on niht ond sing letania ond credan ond pater noster ond writ him cristes mæl on ælcum lime ond nim lytle hand fulle þæs ilcan cynnes wyrta gelice gehalgode ond wyl on meolce, dryp þriwa gehalgodes wætres on ond supe ær his mete, him biþ sona sel.'

'For elf-sickness, take bishopwort, fennel, lupin, the lower part of elfthon, lichen from the hallowed sign of Christ, and storax, take a handful of each, bind up all the plants in a cloth, dip it into hallowed font water thrice, have three masses sung over it-first 'omnibus sanctus', second 'contra tribulationem', third 'pro inwirmis', then put hot coals into a censer, and lay the plants on it; smoke the man with the plants before morning and at night, and sing the litany and the credo and 'pater noster' and mark Christ's sign on each limb, and take a small handful of plants of the same kind, likewise hallowed, and boil them in milk, drip hallowed water in thrice, and let him sip it before his food, it will soon be better for him.'

A further remedy for elf-sickness:

'Eft wiþ þon lege under weofod þas wyrte, læt gesingan ofer viiii mæssan: recels, halig sealt, iii heafod cropleaces, ælfþonan nioþewearde, elenan, nim on morgen scenc fulne meoluce, dryp þriwa haliges wæteres on, supe swa he hatost mæge, ete mid iii snæde ælfþonan ond þonne he restan wille hæbbe gleda þærinne, lege stor ond ælfþonan on þa gleda ond re chine mid þæt he swæte, ond þæt hus geond rec ond georne þone man gesena ond þonne he on reste gange ete iii snæda eolonan, ond

> *iii cropleaces, ond iii sealtes, ond hæbbe him scenc fulne ealað ond drype þriwa haliy wæter on, besupe ælce snæd, gereste hine siþþan, do þis viiii morgenas, ond viiii niht, him biþ sona sel.*

> 'Again, lay these plants under the altar, have nine masses sung over them: incense, holy salt, three heads of cropleek, the lower part of elfthon, elecampane, take a cupful of milk in the morning, drip holy water in thrice, let him sip it as hot as he can, let him eat with it three slices of elfthon and when he wishes to rest let him have coals therein, lay storax and elfthon onto the coals, and steam him with it so that he may sweat and let it steam throughout the house, and sign the man earnestly, and when he goes to his rest let him eat three morsels of elecampane, and three of cropleek and three of salt and let him have a cupful of ale and drip holy water into it thrice, let him swallow each morsel and let him rest himself afterwards, do this for nine mornings and nine nights, it will soon be better for him.'

Healing remedies against elves fell from favour after the Anglo-Saxon period when demons begin to take over where the elves disappeared. Belief in elves did not completely dissipate, however, especially in the more Celtic regions of Britain. In Scotland and Northern England elves still caused havoc for centuries to come and their antics are recorded within the confessions of witches as late as the sixteenth century. There is an intriguing Scottish case where the accused woman, a folk-healer named Bessie Dunlop, allegedly met with a ghost who wanted her to go with him to Elfame. Although the account was delivered during Bessie's trial for witchcraft and therefore cannot be reliable, the story nonetheless contains the common beliefs of the time.

Elves were thought to shape-shift within our world into loved ones or those who were familiar. The ghost that appeared to Bessie was that of Thomas Reid, who had died some years earlier during a battle. He urged Bessie to accompany him to Elfame. Bessie described him as:

> '*ane honest, wele, elderlie man, gray bairdit, and had ane gray coitt with Lumbart slevis of the auld fassoun; ane pair of gray brekis and quhyte schankis gartanit abone the knee; ane blak bonet on his heid, cloise behind and plane befoir, with silkin laissis drawin throw the lippis thairof; and ane quhyte wand in his hand.*'

Thomas introduced her to the '*gude wychtis that wynnit* (dwelt) *in the court of Elfame*'. Bessie was taught many aspects of magic and healing by the elves and fairies and was party to a number of their rituals, whether she cared for it or not. Yet Bessie was loyal to her family and did not wish to go and live in Elfame. Perhaps she should have. She was burnt on Edinburgh's Castle Hill in 1576.

There are many accounts of women being pursued by elves from Elfame and some of the accounts are lively and full of details. The trial of Alesoun Peirsoun (Alison Pearson) in 1588 was even more vivid in its descriptions of a poor young woman plagued by elves who would not take no for an answer. The elves would constantly torment her. She described how they arrived in the wind – 'for they are ever in the blowing sea-wind' – to instruct her in the elvish ways of herbs and healing. Alison became so adept at folk-healing that the Bishop of St Andrews, a hypochondriac, called upon her for remedies. When Alison's cousin returned from abroad, however, he discovered that she was extremely ill and of 'feeble' mind as Alison, he observed, was suffering from seizures, fevers and hysterics. Alison was burnt at the stake in 1588.

The healing principles of our ancestors seem very different from the treatments and drugs available to us today. Yet there are certain commonalties of experience that help to further elucidate the Old English folk-healing tradition. For example, had one suffered from a scaly, itchy rash in the past, a folk-healer may have prescribed, 'goose-fat, and the lower part of elecampane and viper's bugloss, bishop's wort, and cleavers,' to be 'pound… together well, squeeze them out, and add a spoonful of soap. Add a little oil, then mix it thoroughly.' After dispensing the ointment into a small leather pouch, the patient would have left with the instructions to:

> 'lather it on at night. Scratch the neck after sunset, and gently pour the blood into running water, spit three times upon it and say, "Take this disease and depart with it." Go back to the house by an open road, and go in silence.'

Today, a similar skin complaint may elicit a similar response. A prescription of topical ointment such as coal-tar paste or calcipotriol, or even a combination of different creams with complimentary active agents is probable. These modern creams have various properties. For example, they act to moisturise the skin similarly to goose-fat, and calm inflammation like the herb cleavers. I would hope my local general practitioner would avoid recommending blood-letting or spitting three times, but some ritual adherence such as applying the ointment at certain times of day for a particular length of time would be expected. In this particular remedy, the skin complaint is termed *blæco* and the Bosworth-Toller Old English dictionary translates this as leprosy. In eleventh century England leprosy was particularly rampant and had been for some time.

Furthermore, the causes of many illnesses are viewed similarly today. We understand that bacteria and viruses attack their host, infecting the body. Antibiotics are used to wage a war, killing the invasive pathogen and although we do not create a narrative to mythologise this process today, our ancestors with their elves and supernatural creatures achieved a similar aim. They viewed illness as being caused by outside agents thought to be alive. Without knowing about bacteria, these agents were viewed as supernatural identities requiring an equally supernatural response to thwart them. The Old English folk-healing tradition thus exposes an adversarial relational element within its understanding of illness.

Our ancestors saw disease as either a negotiation or war with another being and this relational quality has not entirely disappeared from our contemporary experience. Today we sometimes believe certain illnesses are communicating with us. The common cold might be advising that we are 'run down' and need to take better care of ourselves. Perhaps a succession of colds will tell us to make some differences to our lifestyle. Many other illnesses seem equally informative with their own personal message to deliver; we are eating too much sugar, we are drinking too much alcohol, we need exercise or we require greater rest. We often feel therefore, that we are somehow responsible for our illness. Our ancestors believed similarly, often believing they had angered the gods, spirits or elves into cursing them with disease.

Pliny wrote that the British had a particular habit of leaving offerings when they harvested herbs for healing. Bread was the most common object given to the spirits of the plant, in the hope that the gift would appease them. Fear of angering spirits and elves was a real concern.

This supernatural-pathology is shared by many indigenous cultures. The Amazonian Shuar tribes also believed for example, that little arrows fired by otherworldly spirits caused disease. These arrows, called tsentsak, carried the energy of the malevolent spirit to infect the victim, much akin to a poisoned dart. To extract the venom, the Shuar healer performed rituals to transfer the poison from the arrows into themselves and then out again into a flowing stream to be purified of the malicious intent. Although the Shuar were thousands of miles away from the Old English folk-healers, there is a similarity of belief.

The Old English folk-healing tradition was one of pharmacological herbal ingredients combined with auxiliary psychological and superstitious factors to provide a holistic mind-body intervention. Although the herbal constituents of many remedies are today considered efficacious, the superstitious and ritualistic aspects such as elves and the consideration of days of power are thought to be mere nonsense. We are just beginning to see, however, that these seemingly irrational practices and beliefs were not just superstition but rather, they formed part of an early psychological landscape where healing was more than just a physiological event.

Chapter 4

Raven's Eye

'Wiþ aswollenum eagan genim cucune hræfne, ado þa eagan of on deft cucune gebring on wætre ond do þa eagan þam men on sweoran þe him þearf sie, he wyl sona hal.'

'For swollen eyes, take a raven before it is dead, remove its eyes before it is dead, bring it into water and put the raven's eyes on the nape of the neck of he who is in need, he will soon heal.'

(Bald's *Leechbook III*)

The raven has a rich folkloric tradition. The first bird sent by Noah to find land following the flood, the raven was a symbol of keen sight and second sight. Odin also sent his ravens Huginn (thought) and Muninn (memory) out over the land to report back to him with the knowledge they had gained. It is even told that Odin himself shapeshifted into a raven's form.

Belief in the power of the raven continues today. In the heart of London six ravens guard the Tower where legend states that, 'If the ravens leave the Tower, the kingdom will fall'. So strong is the belief in this superstition that the Tower even keeps a seventh raven in reserve, just in case.

The above remedy for swollen eyes is a prime example of Old English sympathetic healing. Sympathy refers to the principle that similar objects share energetic connections whereby like is attracted by like. This sympathy, or likeness, can then be exploited for healing purposes so that what is done to one thing, will necessarily happen to its corresponding sympathetic partner. This notion is the basis of modern homeopathy yet, in the context of Old English medicine, it is commonly perceived to be a magical principle.

To cure swollen eyes, we are told to 'put the raven's eyes on the nape of the neck of he who is in need'. Today we know that a major artery leads from the nape of the neck to the eyes and although it seems unlikely that this would have been commonly known to our ancestors, it may have been simple observation that led folk-healers to realise a connection between the neck and eyes, as eyestrain and neck ache can manifest together.

The principle of sympathy is clear, linking in corresponding likeness the eye of the raven to that of the human patient. Yet where the raven's eye is keen and healthy, the patient's eye is not, so this cure aims to appropriate the health from the raven's eye to relieve the swelling. This is possibly why, unusually, the prescription is for the eye to be taken from a live bird.

A number of leechbook remedies prescribe the use of ravens. The following one, also for eyes, is less morbid, as one may assume the raven is dead on this occasion, before the extraction of its bile:

> *'Gif eagan forsetene beoð. Genim hræfnes geallan ond hwitmæringe, wudulehtric ond leaxes geallan, do tosommne, dryp on ðæt eage þurh linhæwenne clað ond gehwæde arodes woses, þonne wacað þæt eage.'*
>
> 'If the eyes be blocked, take raven's gall and white maring, wood-lettuce and salmon's gall, put them together, drop it into that eye through blue linen cloth and a small amount of strong juice, then wakens the eye.'

White maring is thought to be sweet basil according to Cockayne when he first translated these manuscripts. The colour of the linen cloth is debatable, as *hæwenne* is a general term describing a variety of strong colours such as blue, green and purple and so possibly refers to a particular pigment used within each. Generally, *hæwenne* is translated as blue as this was considered an auspicious colour by the Anglo-Saxons. *Hæwenne* recurs in further remedies for eye pain and earache.

Sweet basil has anti-inflammatory properties and bile has been used in medicine for thousands of years. In their 2014 paper *Therapeutic Uses of Animal Biles in Chinese Medicine*, Wang and Carey found there are numerous health benefits that can be attributed to bile, including the healing of delicate skin. So, it is conceivable that this remedy may have had some benefit for sore or injured eyes. There is simply no reason today, however, for bile to be harvested from animals. Synthetic and herbal alternatives exist.

Sympathy, used in the context of ritual, is a relatively modern term coined by James Frazer in his classic work *The Golden Bough* (1890). Through observation, Frazer identified and extracted the theory of what he first called sympathetic magic from earlier notions of imitation and contagion. He identifies two traits of sympathetic magic – the law of similarity and the law of contact. These 'laws' exist in contemporary popular culture as the Law of Attraction which mingles, albeit dubiously, with quantum mechanics. The Law of Attraction is based upon the enduring Platonist theory that like attracts like, with modern proponents arguing that quantum physics now offers scientific evidence for this previously magical process.

Although care is needed when referring to quantum physics, as it is currently being used to spuriously evidence numerous psychic, spiritual and New Age phenomena, it does nonetheless share many cosmological philosophic principles with the subject in hand. Einstein certainly speculated that he believed there was 'something' which could travel faster than the speed of light in an attempt to explain why it is that one particle knows at distance what is happening to its other half and changes accordingly without material intervention. But can this particle entanglement really de-mystify the paranormal and bring magic into the realm of science? Probably not or at least, not yet. Our understanding of quantum effect is in its infancy and there is much work to do before anyone could state with certainty that a raven's eye has any curative effect beyond that of a placebo. The mystery of sympathetic magic therefore remains.

Magic was a very real phenomenon for our ancestors and placebo or not, it continues to be used by people today. The spiritual teacher Robbyne La Plant explains and describes magic on her website 'White Wolf Journeys':

> 'Magic is finding your connection to the Earth and all that is natural, alive and moving in the universe! It binds all that exists together. Magic is living in balance with the flow of life, and knowing that you are a vital force within that flow. Magic is everywhere! In the trees, rain, stars, and in the sea. It is the spark that quickens a seed to rise up from the soil. Magic is laughter, joy, wonder and truth of the world around us! It is the subtle enchantment that reminds us not to waste a single moment of this gift that we call life! Magic is not greed, or power, or pretense … It is real. It exists. And it works. Magic is the mystery that lies in the secret soul of the world. It is the essence of creation. What we imagine, we have the power to create! MAGIC IS WITHIN YOU... With it you can create your dreams, heal your world, love your life and find the peace that lives in every human heart.'

La Plant describes magic as an essential human experience that exists as an energy linking everything together. Magic is therefore active, creative and importantly, meaningful. Historian Richard Kieckhefer also views magic as an experiential quality of daily life. From his extensive study of the great Nordic sagas he has found that our ancestor's understanding of magic was central to their very existence and that their stories:

> 'depict magic as occurring amid realistic accounts of everyday situations: in the thick of family feuds, in the exercise of judicial business, in the ordinary grind of life, not in a fantasy world or an idealized or enchanted realm.'
>
> (*Magic in The Middle Ages*, 2011)

Woodcuts from the Middle Ages depicting common folk selling wind-strings to sailors, offer further examples of the belief in sympathetic magic. A wind-string refers to a length of cord with a series of knots tied into it, each knot identifying sympathetically with a different strength of wind. There would be one knot for a gentle breeze, a second for a strong wind and a further knot for a gale. The practitioner would have enabled this sympathetic correspondence through Frazer's further principle of contact. For example, taking the string to a place where the desired strength of wind could be found and, through adjurations, invoking gods old and new, the first knot would be formed in contact with the breeze. The same would then follow for each further knot, which would be created in contact with the corresponding force of wind.

When at sea, the ship's captain would untie the knot for the strength of wind he desired. The earlier contact, secured by intent, would then be released to attract its like. Wind strings relied therefore, on a balance between similarity and contact.

The weather was of great concern to our ancestors and it continues to be an almost obsessive preoccupation of the British today. This is likely due to the geographic position of the country which is located at a point on the globe where competing weather systems are the norm. This makes it almost impossible to predict the weather with any degree of certainty and this lack of predictive capacity can lead to a feeling of helplessness and lack of control. Similarly to healthcare, this lack of control over a phenomenon that appears chaotic and random elicited a supernatural response designed to alleviate fear and helplessness.

A further example of sympathetic magical thinking comes from Bald's *Leechbook III* and concerns a remedy for a cyst or tumour. The cure relies upon the creation of a conceptual relationship between an exterior object such as water evaporating from a bucket, and the desired outcome of annihilation for the cyst. So as the water evaporates, the cyst, now linked in a sympathetic relationship with the water due to the folk-healer's intent, also diminishes to nothing. Here is the full remedy followed by a poetic translation by Gavin Chappel:

'Wenne, wenne, wenchichenne,
her ne scealt þu timbrien, ne nenne tun habben,
ac þu scealt north eonene to þan nihgan berhge,
þer þu hauest, ermig, enne broþer.
He þe sceal legge leaf et heafde.
Under fot wolues, under ueþer earnes,
under earnes clea, a þu geweornie.
Clinge þu alswa col on heorþe,
scring þu alswa scerne awage,
and weorne alswa weter on anbre.
Swa litel þu gewurþe alswa linsetcorn,
and miccli lesse alswa anes handwurmes hupeban,
and alswa litel þu gewurþe þet þu nawiht gewurþe.'

'Wen [cyst], wen, little wen,
Here you shall not build, nor have your abode,
But you shall go north to the hill nearby
Where, benighted one, you have a brother.
He shall lay a leaf at your head.
Under the wolf's foot, under the eagle's wing,
Under the eagle's claw, may you wane forever.
Shrivel like a coal on the hearth,
Shrink like slime on the wall,
Waste away like water in a bucket.
Become as little as a grain of linseed,
and much smaller than a hand-worm's hip-bone,
and so very small that you become nothing.'

Ritual combined with an authoritative performance is used here to set the scene telling the story of the cyst's imminent demise. This is in effect a form of exorcism (of the cyst) and as such may have had a powerful effect upon the patient. Quite sufficient, one might imagine, to provide a belief strong enough to trigger a healing response.

A placebo effect, however, can work both ways. In *Anglo-Saxon Mythology, Migration & Magic* (1994), Tony Linsell suggests that the above remedy for a cyst is not as curative as it may first appear. Rather, he suggests, it is the remnant of a curse reformed as a cure. Although we can never be certain of this, he does present a further, very similar, remedy discovered in a fragment of manuscript from the British Library, which does appear to be a curse and which uses the same sympathetic principles to diminish the unwanted object:

> 'May he quite perish, as wood is consumed by fire, May he be as fragile as a thistle. He who plans to drive away these cattle or to carry off these goods.'

The object intended to be 'consumed by fire' is identified, by the use of the personal pronoun 'he', as a human being. The Oxford English Dictionary defines a curse as, 'A solemn utterance intended to invoke a supernatural power to inflict harm or punishment on someone or something,' and there is an obvious intention in this remedy to cause harm. Yet the harm only occurs in response to a person planning to steal cattle and other goods and so, arguably, this remedy could equally be understood as a protective device. Cattle rustling was a common problem in England at the time as cows were of great value. Taking pro-active defensive measures to ensure their safety would have been of great importance. A curse like this may well have been written down and turned into a protective talisman and nailed to an enclosure as a deterrent against thieves.

The cure for the cyst may therefore have been adaptable. Used as a powerful therapeutic intervention to exorcise a tumour, it could also be suitable for pre-emptive protection against threats generally. A step further and it might transform into a tool of retribution. This is a slippery slope where a more sinister element arises when the curse stands alone in the darker recesses of man's intent.

Protection from disease, harm and theft was an invaluable necessity for our ancestors. Amulets and talismans were used as protective devices carried upon the person, hung on doors and boundaries or buried in the home. Amulets, which were normally created using natural substances, have long been associated with attracting luck. The rabbit's foot is a prime example of this type of charm. Talismans, which include some artificial intervention such as writing, carving or combinations of natural ingredients, were usually used for protecting property and people from illness, theft or any other manner of harm. One such talisman that the scribes assumed was also to ward off thieves is documented in the *Lacnunga* manuscript:

> *'Wið þeofentum, luben luben niga efið niga efið fel ceid fel ceid, delf fel cumer orcggaei ceufor dard giug farig pidig delou delupih.'*

This charm has never adequately been translated. Folklorist Felix Grendon suggests in the *Journal of American Folklore*, that this is an example of what he terms a 'jingle charm,' which is rhythmic, catchy and often nonsensical. There are more such instances within the leechbooks where a seemingly nonsensical string of words, symbols or letters are put together to form a remedy. Some have a metric structure and may have been chanted rather like a mantra or rhyme and Grendon makes the suggestion that many children's nursery rhymes that survive today may be snippets from ancient remedies. For example, a children's counting rhyme from England goes:

> 'Eeny, meeny, miny, mo, catch a tiger by the toe, if he hollers, let him go, eeny meeny, miny, mo.'

This rhyme has evolved from something extremely old and its full meaning is lost. It appears to be based upon an earlier form of Old English than the version that became standard towards the end of the first millennium. It is possible that this might in fact be Old Cornish. Language was slower to change in the more Celtic regions of Britain and in an old form of counting from Cornwall for example, the first four numbers were *eena, mena, mona, mite*. This rhyme may be the remnants of a Cornish healing remedy, it may just as easily be a way of counting sheep in the fields. We may never know.

The *Lacnunga* charm against theft may continue to defy translation but that has not stopped a number of researchers having a go anyway. Lori Ann Garner, for example, thinks it is a very old form of Old Irish and this may be true, but as she concedes, only a few words can be said with any certainty to be Irish. From my own research, I have identified possible etymological links to various Celtic and Old-Germanic dialects that cause me to wonder if this charm is perhaps a transitional language between the Celtic peoples of Britain and Ireland and the Saxon invaders. To arrive at any reasonable translation is therefore difficult, especially, as Grendon has identified, it appears that the last six words are a scribe's attempt to write only two words- *giug farig pidig* are possibly three guesses by the scribe at writing a word which is unfamiliar to him and has not necessarily been written down before, the same may be true for *delou* and *delupih*. The scribe may be hedging his bets regarding these last two words by including a variety of potential spellings, hoping that at least one of them may be correct.

Similarly, the translation of the following snippet from another *Lacnunga* remedy seems equally impossible, '*Acre arcre arnem nona ærnem beoðor ærnem nidren acrun cunað ele harassan fidine.*' It has been suggested by contributors to the Skaldic Project (an academic group bringing together the corpus of Norse and Iceland poetry), however, that this might be a version of Old Norse, although Pollington suggests Celtic scholars have potentially identified the first words as Old Irish meaning 'a charm against blood, against venom'. As the phrase occurs within a larger remedy for a 'holy' salve and holy salves are often protective in nature, then Pollington's theory of blood and poison may be closer to accuracy.

The *Lacnunga* manuscript contains a further remedy against a lump/cyst which relies upon a particularly powerful sympathetic relationship. In the previous cures, we have seen cysts being linked in sympathy with receding water and wood being consumed by fire. In the following remedy the association is particularly impressive, with the tumour's fate allied to that of nine women who, so we are told, are the sisters of *Noðþæs*. The use of the number nine combined with identities of powerful people would have served to amplify the sympathetic nature of this cure to the point where 'every evil' may also be thwarted:

> *'Wið cyrnel, neogone wæran noðþæs sweoster, þa wurdon þa nygone to eahtum, ond eahtai to seofonum, ond þa seofone to sixum, ond sixe to fifum, ond þa fife to feowerum, ond þa feowere to þrim, ond þa þrie to twam, ond þa twa to anum, ond þa an to nanum, þis þe lib beo cyrneles ond scrofelles ond weormes ond æghwylces yfeles, sing benedicite nygon siþum.'*

> 'Against a lump, Nine were Noðþæs sisters, then the nine became eight and the eight to seven, and the seven to six, and the six to five, and the five to four, and the four to three, and the three to two, and the two to one, and the one to none, this shall be the treatment of the lump, and of scrofula, and of a worm and of every evil, sing benedicite nine times.'

The words *Wið cyrnel* seem to be penned in the wrong place in the manuscript. *Cyrnel* means a seed or grain and may be part of the previous remedy. The sympathetic element in this remedy is evident, however, as the lump is likened to the nine sisters of *Noðþæs* who died out one by one. The law of similarity is invoked between the demise of the nine sisters and the tumour or cyst requiring a similar fate. Sympathy is being used here therefore as part of a wider magical process, drawing upon the power of numerology and identities to amplify its effects.

Nine was a very important number to the early Germanic tribes and Celtic peoples alike. We have already seen the importance of the number three. Nine is three times three. This remedy meant business. But who were these nine sisters and their brother? We can assume they were potent figures and according to folklore, there were indeed nine mighty sisters who walked the earth. Tales of them are told from Iceland to the Middle East, in ancient texts and in modern mystery schools and although a small digression is required to investigate these women, their identities are interesting and ultimately, give further indication for whether this cure might also be adaptable as a curse.

There was a Masonic Lodge in Paris in the eighteenth century named The Nine Sisters. In the Rennes archives of Northern France there is also evidence of the existence of nine virgin sisters who lived together on the Ile de Sein, just off the coast from Finisterre, Brittany, near the Pointe du Raz, an area of Brittany that retains many ancient monuments. Carnac for example, not far from the Pointe du Raz, has one the most extensive collection of Neolithic standing stones in the world. The nine sisters of Sein were greatly revered and sought out as healers:

> 'In the Brittanic Sea, opposite the coast of the Ossismi, the isle of Sena (Sein) belongs to a Gallic divinity and is famous for its oracle, whose priestesses, sanctified by their perpetual virginity, are reportedly nine in number. They call the priestesses Gallizenae and think that because they have been endowed with unique powers, they stir up the seas and the winds by their magic charms, that they turn into whatever animals they want, that they cure what is incurable among other peoples, that they know and predict the future, but that it is not revealed except to sea-voyagers and then only to those traveling to consult them.'
>
> (Pomponius, *De Corographia*, 44.C.E.)

The sisters were known to exist into the sixteenth century when, finally, Sein became the last place in Europe and Scandinavia to be converted to Christianity. Due to this, there are contemporaneous descriptions of white-robed priestesses, whose garments covered additional heavier tunics, and who wore conical headdresses similar to, but far taller than, the Brittany headdresses worn on the mainland. Researchers agree that these nine women were druidesses and that they specifically taught the women of the mainland matters of nature and healing. Even today, guidebooks describe the island as holding a mysterious enigmatic quality and that the current inhabitants retain an 'otherness' which includes the celebration of solar rituals.

Within Regino of Prum's *Canon Episcopi* published in the tenth century, it is documented that the Roman Church had great concerns about the Northern European pagan traditions that had still not been wiped out. It particularly mentions that certain women were known to fly through space with the goddesses Diana and Holda, and Carlo Ginzburg argues in *Ecstasies* (1991) that such references indicate 'a primarily female ecstatic religion, dominated by a nocturnal goddess'. Further evidence of a continuing powerful goddess cult in Northern Europe can be seen in the remedy for a sudden stitch that we come to later.

It is probable that these nine sisters or priestesses were the inspiration for the Arthurian legend of Morgan le Fay. Morgan was one of nine sisters, most likely a druid priestess who lived on an enchanted Island. As Thelgesinus tells Merlin in the *Vita Merlini* (1150):

> 'The Isle of Apple Trees, or of Apples is also called 'Blessed Isle' because all its vegetation is natural … The people there live for a hundred years and more. It is ruled by nine sisters under a system of benign laws to which visitors coming from our regions are introduced. Of these nine sisters, one surpasses the others in beauty and power. Her name is Morgen and she teaches the uses of plants and how to cure sickness. She knows the art of changing one's appearance and of flying through the air with the aid of wings, like Daedalus … It is there that, after the battle of Camblan, we took the wounded Arthur on the ship Barintho, guided by the waves and the stars … She had the King carried to a golden couch in her chamber and carefully laid bare his wound. She watched over him for a long time, finally saying that he could recover his health if he remained on the island with her and was willing to accept her treatments.'

It may be the same nine sisters that appear in the welsh poem *Preiddeu Annwfn* from a thirteenth century manuscript called *The Book of Taliesin*. Annwfn is the name given to the Otherworld where Arthur must journey to capture a magical cauldron, (that may be an earlier symbol for what we know today as the holy grail) which, 'from the breath of nine maidens it was gently warmed.'

Turning to their brother, Karl Young concludes in *Anglo-Saxon Charms* (1996), that regarding the *Wið cyrnel* remedy, 'I can't identify Noththes'. Young assumes that Noththes is a personal name, and Griffiths (2006) argues that Noththes is a name meaning boldness or daring and may refer to a character in a story now lost. The surname Noth does exist today and is Germanic in origin, so Griffiths may be correct.

Joseph Frank Payne offers an alternative explanation in his 1902 lecture series on English Medicine in Anglo-Saxon times. He suggests that Noththes may simply refer to a nodal swelling, and that its identification as a person's name could be mistaken.

At the eastern end of Ringstead Bay in Dorset, England, however, there is an outcrop of chalky rock known locally as White Nose, but spelt White Nothe. Nose in Old English is *nosu*, but it is not beyond the imagination to wonder if the ancient West Country accent and dialect caused some confusion that turned *nosu* into *nothe*, the latter of which was committed to ink when the monks began to document these remedies. This theory would be relevant to the utility of the remedy, as *Wið cyrnel* is to be used for a lump or nodule visually similar, perhaps, to the nose. It might be therefore, that Payne is correct and further, that this particular remedy may have been specific to the West Country.

My own research has offered two further alternatives. As *Noðþæs* is specifically mentioned in the cure as being the brother to nine sisters, it seems likely it is indeed a personal name. Given the many scribal errors within the manuscripts indicating a degree of guess work, it might be that *Noðþæs* is a scribal hunch at the name *Níðuðr,* also spelled sometimes as *Niðhad, Niðhades* and *Niðung*. *Níðuðr* is a legendary Germanic King renowned for his power and especially, his cruelty. To invoke such a name and to draw upon the demise of his sisters might enable a very effective remedy or alternately, a particularly powerful curse.

It is also possible that *Noðþæs* refers to the ancient fertility goddess Nerthus or *Nerðþæs*. Evidence of her can be found throughout Germania and Scandinavia and her priestesses, perhaps considered in life to be her sisters, were always nine in number.

Poppet magic was a popular way of using sympathy to perform curses. Although Tony Linsell may be correct in his theory that banishment cures could be curses formed into remedies, the area of sympathetic correspondence where cursing was obvious was when poppets were used. A poppet is a small doll usually made of stone, cloth or wax, created to resemble a person. Often this representation is used for positive intent such as healing and protection, with poppets serving as amulets. The oldest such amulet in the British Isles was discovered in 2009 on the Scottish island of Westray and has been affectionately named the Westray Wifie. The Wifie is 5000 years old, about 4.5 centimetres tall and carved from stone. She is one of a pair found in the remains of a Neolithic village. She wears a checked tunic and bears recognisable facial features, including eyebrows. The figurine was discovered buried within a domestic dwelling.

The custom of leaving female figurines or poppets within houses was common throughout Europe and the Middle East as evidenced by the Venus sculptures, some of which are over 25,000 years old. The oldest undisputed Venus sculpture was discovered near Schelklingen in Germany. She is 6cm tall and made of ivory. Archaeologists date her from between 35,000 to 40,000 years old.

Images of the ancient mother goddess, Ashara, can be found buried in the remains of domestic dwellings all over the Middle East. Professor Judith Hadley argues in her paper *The Cult of Asherah in Ancient Israel and Judah* (2000), that these figurines indicate a very ancient goddess tradition, pre-dating the fragmentation of religious beliefs and culture into Israelite, Canaanite etc. The tree of life or kabala, so commonly associated with the patriarchal Judaic mystery religions, has been postulated to be a symbol for Ashara in pre-Old Testament times. Ashara is mentioned in a number of Hittite and Akkadian texts where she is also known as the Queen of Heaven. We find reference to the Queen of Heaven within The Bible too. In

Jeremiah 7:18, we find the remnants of an ancient ritual to Ashara that included the preparation of bread:

> 'The children gather wood, the fathers light the fire, and the women knead the dough and make cakes of bread for the Queen of Heaven.'

And in Jeremiah 44:15-18:

> 'Then all the men who knew that their wives were burning incense to other gods, along with all the women who were present – a large assembly – and all the people living in Lower and Upper Egypt, said to Jeremiah, "We will not listen to the message you have spoken to us in the name of the LORD! We will certainly do everything we said we would: We will burn incense to the Queen of Heaven and will pour out drink offerings to her just as we and our fathers, our kings and our officials did in the towns of Judah and in the streets of Jerusalem. At that time we had plenty of food and were well off and suffered no harm. But ever since we stopped burning incense to the Queen of Heaven and pouring out drink offerings to her, we have had nothing and have been perishing by sword and famine.'

With so many carvings of Ashara having been placed in the centre of family homes, beneath the hearth, it is considered likely by Hadley that these goddess representations were amulets of protection. The Westray Wifie was also found buried within a home and the Venuses have been unearthed within settlements. Protection for the home, hearth and family seems a likely hypothesis.

Not all poppets were created for such positive purposes. In the year 968, a Scottish king named Duff was wasting away with a mortal illness, which he suspected was the work of diabolical magic. A local family was dragged into the castle where the youngest confessed to the king that there were indeed a number of local folk practicing the dark arts, and that she could tell him where they met. These practitioners of black magic were discovered, rounded up and burnt in Forres in Murray after a waxen image of the king had been recovered. The king had the poppet gently melted and destroyed. His health was regained.

Poppet cursing was not confined to the Dark Ages. In medieval Coventry, a local man involved in a dispute with his neighbour decided to employ magical means to achieve the resolution he desired. He made an image of his neighbour in wax and then hammered a nail through the poppet's head. It is told that the neighbour went completely mad. Not satisfied, the man then drove a second nail through the waxen chest, where the heart would be. This had the desired result, as his neighbour fell down dead.

In 1476, nineteen or so men and women were burnt in Edinburgh for conspiring to create a waxen doll of James III, which they proceeded to roast in flames. A further example occurred in the Middle Ages when a schoolmaster was accused of using a poppet to win the woman he desired. The teacher had paid the young woman's brother to steal three strands of her pubic hair for him to use in a love spell. When the young woman's mother discovered this however, she went out one night to collect three strands of hair from the underside of a cow and told her son to give these to the man as a deception. This he did and, so the story goes, the cow and schoolmaster fell in love and could not be separated. This may seem a fanciful tale until one learns that a poppet within the Boscastle Museum of Witchcraft is fully clothed in every way, right down to its real pubic hair.

Using bodily materials became increasingly popular through the medieval era and in a continental manuscript, we find a particularly unsettling sympathetic remedy attributed to the sixteenth century scientist Gianbattista della Porta. To cure a warrior injured in battle the healer must take:

> 'the moss of an unburied cranium, the fat of a man, each two ounces, mummy, human blood each half an ounce, and linseed oil, turpentine, each one ounce.'

Human fat combined with linseed oil would make a good salve for the injured soldier; however, the ointment must also be applied to the enemy's sword that first caused the injury. The logic being that there is a powerful sympathy between the bloodied object and the injured party, as the spirit or soul exists within their blood. Remedy the blade with such an ointment and the injury should heal. This cure includes human flesh (cranium moss), human fat and human blood. Such ingredients were usually harvested from the recently dead with this method of healing becoming known as corpse medicine.

Chapter 5

Mandrake

'Wyrc sealfe wiþ ælfcynne ond nihtgengan ond þam mannum þe deofol mid hæmð, genim eowohumelan, wermod...'

'Work a salve for elf-kind, and nightgoers, and the people who have sex with the devil, take English mandrake, wormwood ...'
(Bald's *Leechbook III*)

Eowohumelan is English mandrake (also known as White Bryony) and combined with wormwood (*wermod*) makes a potentially dangerous remedy. In large doses, mandrake can kill and wormwood may cause seizures, excessive diarrhoea and death. Interestingly, where mandrake is a soporific, wormwood is a stimulant, so we see once more how a number of the Old English remedies contain seemingly counter-acting ingredients with the opposing actions combining to produce a balanced, sophisticated result in the right quantities.

Mandrake is used in ancient remedies as both a pharmaceutical and ritualistic device. Its role in ritual derives from its resemblance to the human form, a connection thought to be powerfully symbolic and magically useful. Following from the notion of sympathetic correspondences between objects, mandrake also illustrates the other main magical principle found in the more supernatural elements of the remedies, that of transference.

Transference is a familiar term today; known from its use within psychotherapeutic vocabulary, it describes the relational process between a patient and their psychotherapist. For example, a patient who has experienced early childhood trauma, perhaps parental abuse, may in analysis transfer the deep grief, anger and other associated emotions onto the therapist, viewing and reacting to them as they would the absent parent. If the therapist observes this process happening, it offers great insight into the unconscious material that needs to be brought into consciousness to enable psychological healing. Although transference happens all the time, in all relationships both personal and social, as a psychological tool we can literally see ourselves reflected in others and if we can become aware of our own transference, we can explore it, use it and transform ourselves. Sigmund Freud first observed transference occurring within his therapeutic sessions.

The emotions transferred by a patient may be positive as well as negative. Patients sometimes fall in love with their therapist or ascribe to them mystical powers, as Dr Halpert states:

> 'Transference to physicians contains a fantasy of the physician as omnipotent healer who can control life and death.'
> (*Asclepius: magic in transference to physicians*, Oct, 1994).

Therapists may also experience counter transference where their own unconscious associations are triggered and come into play, especially when the wounds of the therapist match the wounds of the patient. None of this is unusual (although Jung believed it could be extremely dangerous). In Freud's *An Autobiographical Study* (1925), he explains the commonality of transference:

> 'It is a universal phenomenon of the human mind, it decides the success of all medical influence, and in fact dominates the whole of each person's relations to his human environment.'

The relational quality of transference underpins its use within Old English healing. Mandrake acts within the remedies as a powerful symbol linking the human patient to the element of earth and the supernatural realm where such likenesses arise. Our ancestors saw mandrake as a real mind-body solution to many of the more psychological remedies, using it for its soporific action and for its uncanny resemblance to the human form. By using this sympathetic likeness, they were able, through ritual, to transfer the illness from a patient into the mandrake thereby affecting healing.

Mandrake is mentioned in ancient texts such as the Bible (where Reuben, the eldest son of Jacob, collects mandrakes for his mother) through to perhaps the most exhaustive recommendations from Saint Hildegard of Bingen (1098-1179) who had a keen interest in Old Germanic folk customs and amassed a wealth of healing materials from the peoples of Northern Europe. Hildegard was a Benedictine Abbess of great renown. Although belittling herself as a weak and unlearned woman, she amassed a wealth of writings on medicine, science and poetry as well as being a competent musical composer and talented artist. From the age of three, Hildegard experienced divine visions, which caused her parents to place her in the enclosure of the Benedictines. Her visions continued and although writing, preaching and teaching were against the Church's recommendations for women of the time, Hildegard said that God had told her to write and share her knowledge. She wrote a large treatise on healing in the twelfth-century called *Physica*, consisting of nine volumes. Bruce Hozaski, who has researched and translated Hildegard's work, suggests that she was not just accumulating previous material, but writing from her own practical experience. Hildegard had moved from copying previous, accepted classical works to collecting healing folk customs of the early Germanic people. She was particularly interested in mandrake, explaining the applications of the herb at some length:

> 'It [is] hot at first … and is formed from the earth from which Adam was made. It looks like a person but is a herb that comes in two forms: one is the man, the other the woman; the form of the woman is somewhat nicer.'

Hildegard's description of mandrake sees it reflecting the human form, which was created from the same substance as Adam. Representing both sexes, the implication is that mandrake and humans have been in relationship from the very beginning, mirroring each other within the genesis myth, forever entwined and interdependent. It is perhaps unsurprising therefore, that one of Hildegard's most detailed remedies has a moral flavour to it, seeking to unburden the patient from lustful desires:

> 'For a man who cannot control himself and is uncouth from sinful ways or from the uncouthness of burning heat, he should take the female form of mandrake, to cleanse it in water, as I have described earlier, and cut from it that which is between the breast and navel … and bind it on his navel for three days and three nights. Then cut the same piece in half and bind a piece on each hip for three days and three nights. Powder also the left hand of the herb, add a small amount of camphor to the powder … and eat it … so his impure desires will be reduced.
>
> 'For a woman who cannot control her uncouthness she should take the herb mandrake, which has the man's form, and work with it in a similar manner to that written before: but the powder should be from the right hand.'

These remedies would certainly have calmed any sensuous desires. Camphor has a depressive action when taken internally and mandrake is intensely soporific so both man and woman would probably have fallen asleep or at the very least, have felt any amorousness seeping away. Hildegard then goes on to list the various healing attributes of mandrake. First, she teaches the importance of sympathy by describing how one should use the part of the root that corresponds to the area of the human body that is hurt. Then follows a short list of disorders specifically remedied by the plant:

> 'It should be known that mandrake is good to use for all trembling. Whoever has a headache, from whichever disorder it comes, he should eat from the head-like part of the herb, however much he wants, it will be reduced … He who has a pain in the throat should eat from the throat and the pain will go

> from him … whatever kind of pain the person has, he should eat of the herb from the place where the similarity lies, it aids his health … Mandrake is good against poison … It is good against disorders of the liver … it is also good against disorders of the loins … disorders of the lungs … It also reduces swelling of the spleen.'

Despite all the beneficial uses mentioned above, Hildegard is careful to make clear the essentially evil nature of Mandrake. Because mandrake root resembles the human body, it may have been seen as the devil's attempt to appear in human form and therefore, present a perversion of Adam or perhaps, Christ. Hildegard thus warns, 'the devil lies therein and his spirit is there … [it] has a great deal of evil with it, as sometimes happens with idols'. She advises therefore that one should:

> 'dig this herb out, and one should throw it into a spring for a day and a night; thus the water takes all evil humours out, so it is therefore no longer good for evil doing. '

Hildegard recommends that mandrake is only viable if it is first purged of evil by the use of water, which would alter it from an implement of malefic magic into a benign herb for healing. We can see how Hildegard links the evil of mandrake to the concept of idols in her *Scivias,* written in 1151:

> 'Those deceived by idols are in the power of perdition, and through idols the unbelievers forsake the honour of their Creator, entangling themselves in the traps of the devil and carrying out his works according to his will.'

Writing a little before the formal establishment of the inquisition in 1232, Hildegard would have been aware of a turning tide in attitudes within the Roman Church towards folk-healing. The *Canon Episcopi* was certainly already in circulation within Germany by the early eleventh century, where it was the first formal Church document to identify folk-healers not just as evil but specifically as female, stating that they were 'wicked women'. It was very important therefore, for Hildegard to situate her passion for folk-healing within a Christian narrative. To accomplish this Hildegard acted much as the Old English monks who transcribed Bald's *Leechbook III* and *Lacnunga* had done before her; she took ancient pre-Christian remedies and translated them into a Christian framework. Similarly to the texts, this process or alteration was not always complete and in in the next remedy discovered by Hildegard, the original healer's beliefs are still evident:

> 'Whoever has a depressed nature or sadness and worry in the heart, he should lay the mandrake which has been cleansed, next to him in bed. So that the mandrake heats up with his sweating, and speak thus; "God, who from the earth made men on earth without pain, I lay now next to me this earth, which has never been corrupted, that my earth also feels joy as you intended." You will then feel the depression leave you and joy fill your heart.'

Here, the mandrake is described in the adjuration as having 'never been corrupted'. This description, which may have gone unnoticed by Hildegard, indicates that there was at one time a more positive relationship with mandrake, where it was viewed as good rather than evil. Hildegard would have been careful to avoid this view as it may have left her vulnerable to unfortunate accusations. Anything that indicated mandrake worship or idolatry was viewed as a heretical belief, challenging not just the notion of original sin but also the verity of the unique nature of Christ. Caution was indeed necessary. The Knights Templar, for example, were accused of worshipping mandrake in the thirteenth century. It is also well documented that common folk held mandrake in high regard and used the roots as amulets to ward off evil and ill fortune. With this lucky and beneficial association, mandrake became quite a challenge to the power of the Church as this journal entry explains:

> 'In 1426 one Friar Richard, of the order of the Cordeliers, preached a fierce sermon against the use of this amulet, the temporary effect of which was so great, that a certain number of his congregation delivered up their "mandragoires" [mandrake amulets] to the preacher to be burnt.'
>
> (*Journal a'un Bourgeois de Paris*, 1429)

In very large doses mandrake can mimic death. Pliny documents it as an ancient anaesthetic used to render a patient unconscious, diminishing signs of life, slowing the heart to extreme bradycardia. As long as the dose was carefully calculated, the deathly state was temporary, although the body could remain in deathly appearance for as long as three days before life miraculously returned. The sleeping potion given by the monk to Juliet demonstrates the effects of such a dose describing that:

> 'When, presently, through all thy veins shall run
> A cold and drowsy humour, which shall seize
> Each vital spirit; for no pulse shall keep
> His natural progress, but surcease to beat:
> No warmth, no breath shall testify thou livest;
> The roses in thy lips and cheeks shall fade
> To paly ashes; thy eyes' windows fall,
> Like death, when he shuts up the day of life;
> Each part, deprived of supple government,
> Shall stiff, and stark, and cold, appear like death.
> Thou shalt remain full two and forty hours
> And then awake as from a pleasant sleep.'

Mandrake's mimicry of death may be the source for the folkloric belief that mandrake will scream when it is pulled from the ground. This is not just any scream, however; this scream will kill anyone that hears it. The origin of this ancient belief is not known although Alice Kuzniar in her 1995 essay *Stones that Stare or the Gorgon's Gaze*, considers it may be part of a continued experience of transference between the plant and mankind where:

> 'The mandrake seems to represent the return of a forgotten, repressed materiality that becomes isolated and embodied in the vengeful scream.'

Due to the deadly consequences of harvesting mandrake, methods were employed to protect human ears from the scream. One technique was to use a dog to pull the root out from the ground. In the Old English *Herbarium* we find the following description regarding the harvesting of mandrake using a dog:

> 'When you come to it, you will know it in that it shines at night like a lantern, when first you see its head, mark round it quickly with iron before it flees, its power is great and so splendid that it will soon escape from an unclean man when he comes towards it, for which reason you mark round it … and you must dig around it so that you do not touch it with the iron but you must vigorously dig up the earth with an ivory wand and when you see its hands and feet, bind them, then take the other end and tie it to a dog's neck, let the dog be hungry, then throw meat before him so he cannot reach it unless he should pull up the plant. Concerning this plant it is told that it has such might that whatever pulls it up will quickly be betrayed in a similar way, whereby as soon as you see that it is drawn up and you have control of it, take it immediately in your hand and twist it and wring the juice from the leaves into a glass vessel.'

There are many herbal illustrations of mandrake being tied to a dog and this practice seems to have been quite normal for over two thousand years. Peter Jones comments in his 1999 facsimile of *Medicina Antiqua* that regarding mandrake:

> 'Pliny repeats the famous story of the dog which pulls it from the ground with the aid of a chain, and perishes in the task, without reservation or comment.'

The Franciscan monk Bartholomew of Suffolk, also known as Bartholomew the Englishman, wrote similarly in his thirteenth century *De proprietatibus rerum* that one should use an iron sword and draw three circles around the mandrake as the sun is setting, otherwise the plant 'slayeth' the man. Josephus informs us, however, that there is another way to harvest the plant, using a type of large mechanical mousetrap which, using a spring mechanism, can pull the root from the ground at a safe distance.

It could be suggested that mandrake's mimicry of the human form has acted as a repository for changing trends regarding how humanity experiences itself. In pre-Christian times the natural world was often honoured, worshipped and experienced as being in an intimate relationship with humanity. During this time, the mandrake seems to have enjoyed a high, uncorrupted status. As Christianity developed, the notion of original sin, specifically focusing upon the inherent evil within women and sex, mandrake, manifesting the likeness of the two sexes, was seen as evil and the folk-healers using it became 'wicked women'. This re-casting of roles in response to changing religious trends could be argued as a meta-transference. Mandrake is rarely used in herbal remedies today. Its magical heritage continues to enliven the imagination, however, as its appearance in the Harry Potter books and films demonstrate. Mandrake may always hold a controversial allure.

Within the Old English folk-healing tradition, we can see transference acting on a number of levels. The ritualistic actions surrounding illness and medical intervention were imbued with meaning and although our ancestor's understanding of transference may lack the complexity born of Freud, transference was used to understand and deal with disease, suffering and fear. A good example of the phenomenon can be found in Bald's *Leechbook*. It is a remedy to help a mother nourish her baby:

> *'Se wifman se ne mæge bearn afedan nime þonne anes bleoos cu meoluc on hyre handa ond gesupe þonne mid hyre muþe ond gange þonne to to yrnendum wætere ond spiwa þærin þa meolc ond hlade þonne mid þære ylcan hand þoμs wæteres muðfulne*

> *ond forwelge, cweþe þonne þas word: "gehwer freed ic me þone mœran magapihtan mis þysse mœran metepihtan þone ic me wille habban ond ham gan.", þonne heo to þan broce ga, þonne ne beseo heo no, ne eft þonne heo þanan ga, ond þonne ga heo in oþer hus oþer he out ofeode ond þœr gebyrge metes'.*
>
> 'For the woman who cannot nourish her child: take the milk of a cow of one colour in her hand, sip up a little with her mouth, and then go to running water and spit the milk into it. And then with the same hand she must take a mouthful of water and swallow it. She is then to say these words "Everywhere I carried with me this strong one, strong because of this great food, such a one I want to have and go home with". When she goes to the stream she must not look round, nor again when she goes away from there, and let her go into another house than the one she started, and there take food.'

The object of transference here is the evil spirit believed to be infecting the woman resulting in her inability to nourish her child. Water acts to take away the spirit after it has been transferred into the milk and spat into the stream. Water also acts to cleanse the woman of any lingering effects when she drinks it. By not looking around, the woman ensures the spirit being carried away in the water could not jump back into her. Going home to a different house would confuse the spirit if it did indeed try to locate her. These are instinctive motivations being moulded into magical ritual.

It has been suggested by Tony Linsell that a cow of just one colour may have been quite rare in Dark Ages England and so the milk from such a cow was perhaps considered to be purer than the milk of a dual coloured cow. Using such a cow's milk as the method of transference may have been symbolically meaningful. There is a similar Old English remedy from the Western MS.46 document that also directs to use the milk from single coloured cow: 'For liver disease, take liverwort; let it be carried home under your knee; boil it in milk from a cow of one colour and mix butter with it'. In *Lacnunga* there is a specific recommendation for a holy salve from a cow, 'of a single colour, so that she be all red or white and unmarked'. Pollington suggests the Old English word for red (read) is mostly likely referring to a tawny brown colour here.

Similarly to the use of poppets in sympathetic magic, transference also has its darker side. Water, milk, herbs and roots are the usual modes of transference yet sometimes, especially when nightwalkers are mentioned, the prescriptions become less straightforward as this curious and unpleasant transference remedy for a persistent headache indicates:

> *'Wiþ swiþe ealdum headfodece....To þon ilcan sec lytle stanas on swealwan bridda magan ond heald þæt hie ne hrinan eorþan ne wætre ne oþrum stanum, beseowa hira iii, on þon þe þu wille do on þone mon þe him þearf sie, him biþ sona sel. Hi beoþ gode wiþ heafodece ond wiþ eagwærce ond wiþ feondes costunga ond nihtgengan ond lencten adle ond maran ond wyrtforbore ond malscra ond yflum gealdorcæftum. Hit sculon beon micle briddas þe þu hie scealt on findan.'*

> 'For a very old headache ... for that find little stones in the stomachs of a swallow's fledglings and hold them so that they do not touch earth nor water nor other stones, sew together three of them in whatever you will, put them on the man to whom they are needful, better he will soon be. They are good for headache, and for eye pain, and for the enemy's temptations, and for nightwalkers, and the spring ailment, and nightmares, and herb craft, and enchantments, and evil witchcraft. It must be in large fledglings that you will find them.'

A number of ailments are included in this remedy; a persistent headache, eye pain and perhaps neurological or psychological issues indicated by the inclusion of symptoms relating to nightwalkers and evil. Such an array of ailments specific to the head and mind might indicate a locus of migraine or brain tumour. Intestinal stones from fledgling swallows are the objects into which the malady is to be transferred. There is an indication that the stones must be put together in a pouch and kept upon the person as an amulet to protect from further symptoms.

One of the least savoury transference remedies I have seen comes from a fifteenth century Italian woman named Matteuccia Francisci who developed a unique cure for lameness. She is known to have brewed together over thirty different herbs whilst singing incantations. When the elaborate potion was ready, the patient was instructed to pour it out into the street so that their lameness would be transferred to the next person to walk along. The remedy was considered to be very effective. Perhaps the worst, however, comes from *Lacnunga*:

> *'Se wifmon se hyre beran afedan ne mæge, genime heo sylf hyre agenes cildes gebyrgenne dæl, wry æfter þone on blace wulle ond bebicge to cepemannum ond cweþe þonne, "ic hit bebicge, ge hit bebicgan þas swearten wulle ond þysse sorge corn."'*

> 'The woman who cannot bear a child, she must take for herself part of her own child's grave, afterwards cover it in black wool and sell it to traders and then say, "I sell it, you buy it, this blackened wool and this sorrowful seed".'

Stillbirths or miscarriage were probably the issue here. The solution, however, is unpleasant to say the least. Death itself is the object being transferred or 'sold' to the unwitting traders. It is unclear whether the 'part' of the dead child's grave refers to the dirt, burial items or even the child itself. The latter may sound gruesome, but using pieces of corpse was not altogether unusual. Matteuccia Francisci used baby bones for one of her sympathetic remedies which was considered to be a good general tonic for all manner of illness. It directs the patient to take:

> 'a bone from an unbaptised baby out to a crossroad, burying it there, and saying various prayers and formulas on that spot over nine days.'

Using body parts such as the bones of a child was a common prescription well into relatively modern times. Christopher Irvine (1620-93) was a respected physician and doctor to King Charles II, and he believed strongly in the transference of spirits as a cure for disease. The four Hippocratic humours (two forms of bile, phlegm and blood) were thought to be full of human spirit, so remedies were often imbued with human sweat, bile, blood, tissues and bones. Irvine cautioned against contact with unhealthy people as this could cause the sick spirits of that person to transfer to the healthy human being.

Here we can see the evolution of medical understanding. Irvine's belief that spirit resides in the body and that this spirit may transfer disease to others is an understanding of infection at a time when germs were yet to be discovered. Irvine does not talk of elves, goblins or nightwalkers and in the seventeenth century he would have been ridiculed for doing so, but his notion of indwelling spirit or essence achieves a similar end nonetheless. Medical and psychological understanding continues to evolve, often with the past falling victim to the ridicule and incredulity of the present.

Chapter 6

Remedy for Sudden Stitch and The Nine Herbs Charm

Wið færstice (for a sudden stitch) is one of the more elaborate remedies we find in the texts and uses the principles of sympathy and transference combined with the further healing devices of singing and dramatization. Singing does not mean the religious chanting or invocation known in contemporary religions but refers to a level of poeticism and story weaving in the ancient remedies that elevated the common word into something far more evocative. Song was power. Poets and singers were often shamanic figures in Anglo-Saxon England known as *woðbora*, literally song-bearer, although *woþ* or *woð* also means inspiration, which is a clue to the role of the singer as healer. The healer would use a singing narrative to induce a trance-like state to contact otherworldly beings. This would be combined with narcotics and sometimes dance.

One example of this can be found in a small cure to remedy what the Anglo-Saxons called 'water-elf sickness', although it remains unclear exactly what water-elf sickness really is. I have seen it argued as a variety of ailments from dysentery to chickenpox. The symptoms and context of the remedy indicate to me that it is something to do with blood loss, or sepsis following a wound:

> *'Gif mon biþ on wæterælfadle þonne him þa handnæglas wonne ond þa Eagan tearige ond wile locian niþer, do him þis to læcedome: eoforþrote, caauc, fone nioþoweard, eowberge, elehtre, eolone, merscmealwan crop, fenminte, dile, lilie, attorlaþe, polleie, murubie, docce, Ellen, felterre, wermod,*

streawbergean leaf, consoled, ofgeot mid ealaþ, do halig wæter to, sing þis gealdor ofer þriwa: Je binne awrat, betest beadowræda, swa benne ne burnon, ne burston, ne fundian ne feologan, ne hoppetan, ne wund Waco sian, ne dolh diopian, ac him self healed hale wæge, ne ace þe þon ma þe eorþan on eare ace. Sing þis manegum siþum: eorþe þe on bere ealle hire mihtum ond magenum; þas galdor mon mæg singan on.'

'If someone should be in water-elf sickness then his fingernails will be paile, and eyes watery and he will look downwards. Do this for him as a leechdom – take boarthroat, hassock, the lower part of Iris, yewberry, lupin, a sprig of marshmallow, fen mint, dill, lily, atterloathe, pennyroyal, horehound, dock, dwarf elder, felter, wormwood, strawberry leaf, comfrey, pour with ale, add blessed water. And sing this charm over it thrice – "I wreathed the wound, best of battle bandages, so injuries should not burn, nor burst, nor spread, nor fade, nor throb, nor the wound be weak, nor the scar deepen, but keep for itself the blessed vessel, nor ache any more than earth would ache in the ear." Sing this many times – "May Earth bear you up with all her powers and might." These charms one may sing onto the wound.'

An interesting aspect of this charm is its structure. First, we see an account of the symptoms the health practitioner should look for such as watery eyes and pale nails. Following this is a list of herbs needed for the medicinal aspect of the remedy. Next, we have the magical application, which involves the healer asserting their power over the evil spirit in song. There is talk of a battle and a wound which the healer has bound to ensure that the 'wound be not weak' or 'any scar deepen'.

The telling of the tale of the illness, and the commanding position of the person exorcising the spirit are common to Old English cures. Following this there is a protective element to the remedy that is also sung. In this case, it invokes the protection of Mother Earth herself. Sometimes these singing aspects can take on a high degree of poeticism. The idea that a poetic declaration establishes power and authority is ancient. It's also found in the troubadour tradition of the Catalan region for example, where even conflicts were fought through the performance of poems and song. The next remedy called *Wið færstice* (For a sudden stitch/pain) contains all these elements:

'Wið færstice: feferfuige ond seo reade netele, ðe þurh ærn nwyxð, ond wegbrade; wyll in buteran.
"Hlude wæran hy, la! hlude ða hy ofer þone hlæw ridan, wæran anmode ða hy ofer land ridan.
Scyld ðu ðe nu, þu ðysne nið genesan mote.
Ut, lytel spere, gif her inne sie!
Stod under linde, under leohtum scylde, þær ða mihtigan wif hyra mægen beræddon, ond hy gyllende garas sændan; ic him oðerne eft wille sændan, fleogende flane forane togeanes.
Ut, lytel spere, gif hit her inne sy!
Sæt smið sloh seax, lytel iserna wundrum swiðe.
Ut, lytel spere, gif her inne sy!
Syx smiðas sætan, wælspera worhtan.
Ut, spere, næs in, spere!
Gif herinne sy isernes dæl, hægtessan geweorc, hit sceal gemyltan.
Gif ðu wære on fell scoten, oððe wære on flæsc scoten, oððe wære on blod scoten, oððe wære on lið scoten, næfre ne sy ðin lif atæsed; gif hit wære esa gescot, oððe hit wære ylfa gescot ond oððe hit ære hægtessan gescot, nu ic wille ðin helpan.
Þis ðe to bote esa gescotes, ðis ðe to bote ylfa gescotes, ðis ðe to bote hægtessan gescotes, ic ðin wille helpan.
Fleoh þær on fyrgen holt, fyrtst ne heafde.
Hal westu nu, helpe ðin drihten."
Nim þonne þæt seax, ado on wætan.'

'[Take] feverfew and the red nettle that grows through a house. And plantain, boil in butter.
"Loud were they, lo, loud! when they rode over the barrow, They

were determined when they rode over the land.
Shield now thyself, so you may survive this attack.
Out little spear, if thou be herein.
[I] stood under linden, under a light shield, Where the mighty women made ready their powers,
And yelling they sent spears.
I will send another back to them, a flying arrow in opposition to them.
Out little spear, if it be herein.
A smith sat, forged a knife; [small the iron, mighty the wound].
Out little spear, if it be herein.
Six smiths sat, wrought slaughter-spears.
Out spear, be not in, spear.
If herein be a bit of iron, work of hags, it shall melt. If you were shot in the skin, or were shot in the flesh, or were shot in the blood, or were shot in the bone,
or were shot in the limb, never may your life be threatened.
If it were the god's shot, or it were the elves shot, or it were the hags shot, I shall now help you.
This is to you a remedy for esa shot, This is to you a remedy for elves shot,
This is to you a remedy for hags shot, I will help you.
It fled to the mountain.
Whole be now, may the Lord help you."
Then take the knife, apply the potion.'

The medicinal element of this charm is straightforward. The herbs stated at the beginning – feverfew, red nettle and plantain – are to be boiled in butter to produce a salve or ointment. Feverfew and plantain, when applied topically, relieve inflammation and red nettle was used to poultice wounds and stop the bleeding. Following this, however, we have quite a story about an attack from otherworldly spirits, 'Loud were they, Lo, Loud!' It's almost like the beginning of Beowulf. It's a strong announcement designed to take control and show the spirit who is in charge.

Next, we are told the story of the infection. The remedy refers to mighty women, hags, smiths, elves and spears. The mighty women are likely the nine sisters or even the Valkyrie, riding out through the fields of battle, or perhaps they are part of the great wold hunt of Herla, King of the ancient Britons. The narrative is interspersed with the phrase, 'Out little spear, if thou be herein,' and this acts as a focused mantra, commanding the otherworldly spears to leave the patient. This specific repetition makes it likely that the remedy is a cure for a range of illnesses that the Anglo-Saxons believed were due to arrows or spears from creatures such as elves and hags. The term hags-shot is still used colloquially in Germany to describe rheumatism, although the inclusion of *esa* (gods) within the remedy indicates this is perhaps intended as a general cure all.

The healer declares that she has special protection from standing beneath the lindenwood tree in a circle of light energy. We are then told of the virtue of the knife, a tool forged by six smiths (a multiple of three) that will be used to apply the powerfully charged salve at the conclusion of the ritual. Then follows a list of all possible evildoers, including hags, elves and the ills they may have caused. The healer claims mastery over all the ailments and states that the remedy will certainly help. She then casts the evil ones to a mountain and protects the patient with the salve applied with the knife of power. *Wið færstice* is probably one of the most complete and coherent Anglo-Saxon remedies that exists today. Many other charms may once have been just as elaborate.

Controversy surrounds the next remedy from *Lacnunga*. The Nine Herbs Charm (note the further multiples of three) as it has been named often stands alone as an object of research and has received the most interest from academics. It retains a large amount of ritualistic material as well as rare mentions of pre-Christian deities. The remedy appears to have been rather garbled in its transcription, with the scribe perhaps assuming it to be just another remedy, specifically, a cure for snakebite. There is evidence of corruption, and changes in the form of later Christianisation, but the curiosities that remain have led historian and psychologist Brian Bates to suggest that this remedy includes the remnants of an ancient, now lost, initiation rite. It is a compelling theory and a historically important one if correct. One thing is evident – this is not just a herbal remedy and it certainly isn't a cure for snakebite.

When first reading the Nine Herbs Charm, the controversy surrounding it seems rather strange. It is structurally similar to the cure for a sudden stitch and seems therefore, somewhat familiar. We are introduced to certain herbs and their healing power followed by a great story concluded by the taking of otherworldly power by the healer. Yet within the charm we find some curious verses such as these:

> 'A snake came crawling, it tore apart a man.
> For Woden took nine glory-twigs,
> he smote the adder that it flew apart into nine parts.
> There the Apple accomplished it against poison
> that she [the serpent] would never dwell in the house.
>
> Chervil and Fennell, two very mighty one,
> They were created by the wise Lord, holy in heaven as He hung;
> He set and sent them to the seven worlds,
> to the wretched and the fortunate, as a help to all.'

The first line has caused many researchers and the original scribes to conclude that this is a cure for snakebite. However, a very early spelling mistake turned one small word spelt in Old English as *nan* into *man*, and almost every person following who relied upon that translation includes the same mistake in their own research. The mistaken translation therefore states that the snake bit a man, *toslat he man*, yet when the text is consulted it reads that the snake bit none, *toslat he nan*. This matches a later line where a worm/snake comes crawling, yet again causes no harm. So, if the snake doesn't bite anyone, something else may be going on. Before delving deeper, however, here is the charm in full. Its Old English version can be found in Appendix One:

REMEDY FOR SUDDEN STITCH . . .

'Remember, Mugwort, what you made known,
What you arranged at the Great proclamation.
You were called Una, the oldest of herbs,
you have power against three and against thirty.

You are mighty against poison and against disease,
you have power against the loathsome foe roving through the land.
And you, Plantain, herbs mother,
Open from the east, mighty inside,
over you chariots creaked, over you queens rode,

over you brides cried out, over you bulls snorted.
You withstood them all, and crashed against them.
May you withstand poison and infection
and the hateful foe roving through the land.
Crash is the name of this herb, it grew on a stone,

it stands up against poison, it dashes against pain.
Nettle it is called, it withstands against poison.
It drives out the hostile one, and casts out poison,
This is the herb that fought against the snake,
it has power against poison, it has power against infection,

she stands against the hateful foe going through the land.
Put to flight now, Viper's Bugloss, the greater poisons,
The nightmare is the lessened, until you have the advantage,
Be mindful, Chamomile, what you made known,
what you accomplished at Alorforda,

that never a man should lose his life from infection
after Chamomile was prepared for his food.
This is the herb that is called wergulu,
A seal sent it across the sea-right,
a vexation to poison, a help to others.

These nine have power against nine poisons.
A snake came crawling, it tore nothing.
Then Woden took nine glory-twigs,
he smote the serpent that it flew apart into nine parts.
There the Apple accomplished it against poison

that she [the serpent] would never dwell in the house.
Chervil and Fennell, the mighty two.
They were created by the wise Lord,
holy in heaven as He hung;
He set and sent them to the seven worlds,

to the wretched and the fortunate, as a help to all.
It stands against pain, it dashes against poison,
it has power against three and against thirty,
against the hand of a fiend and against noble devices,
against the charm of vile creatures.

Now these nine herbs have power against nine evil spirits,
against nine poisons and against nine infections:
Against the red poison, against the foul poison.
against the white poison, against the blue poison,
against the yellow poison, against the green poison,

against the dark poison, against the blue poison,
against the brown poison, against the red poison.
Against worm-blister, against water-blister,
against thorn-blister, against thistle-blister,
against ice-blister, against poison-blister.

Against harmfulness of the air, against harmfulness of the ground, against harmfulness of the sea.

If any poison comes flying from the east,
or any from the north, [or any from the south,]

A facsimile of a page from Bald's *Leechbook*.

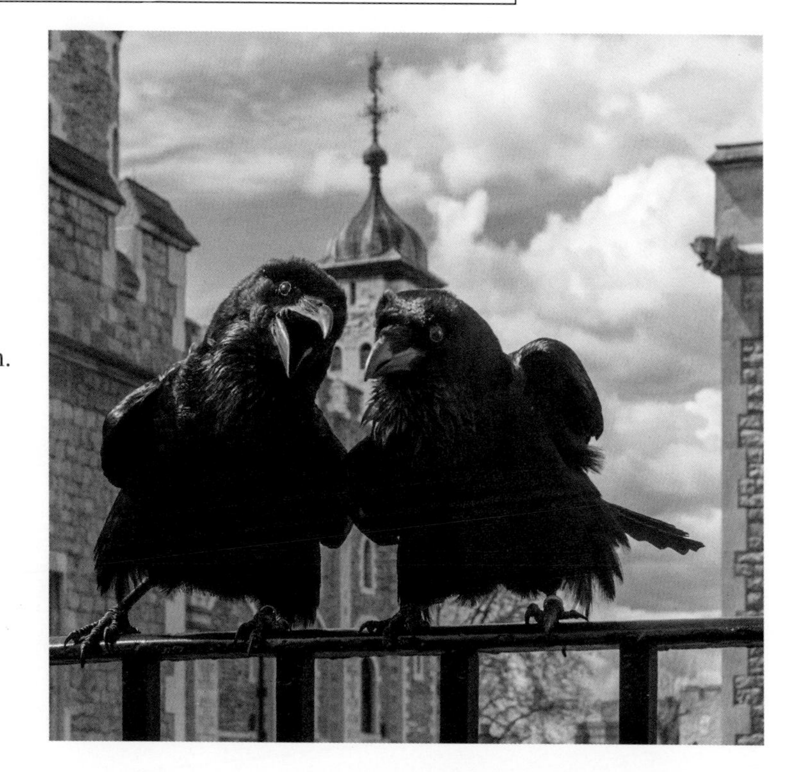

Odin and Thor, ravens, at the Tower of London.

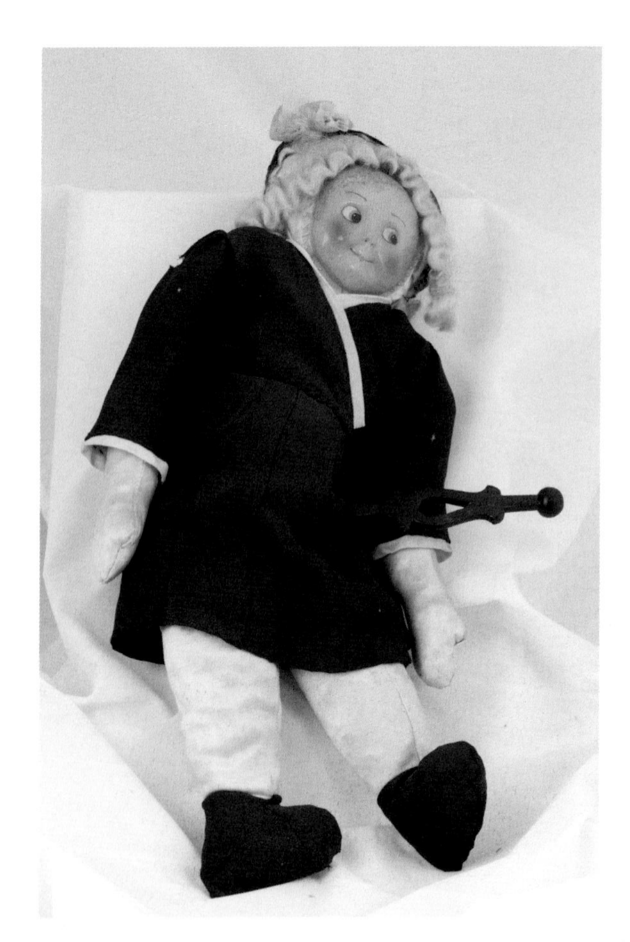

Poppet used in image magic. (Image copyright Museum of Witchcraft & Magic, Boscastle.)

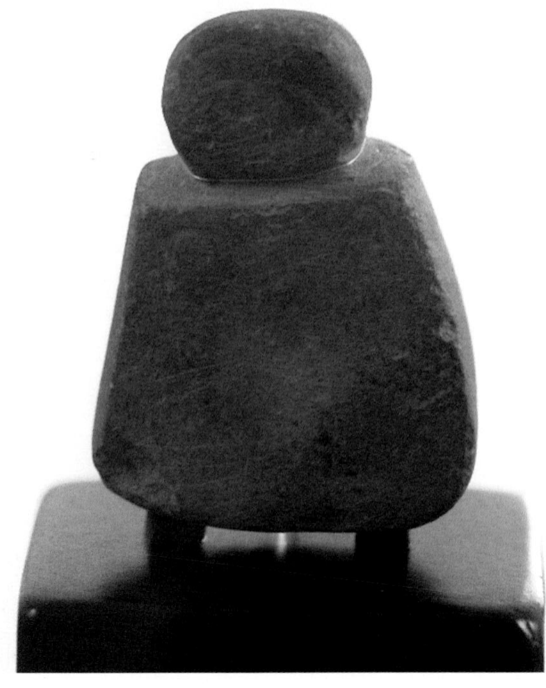

Westray Wife, found on the Links of Noltland, Westray, Orkney, Scotland.

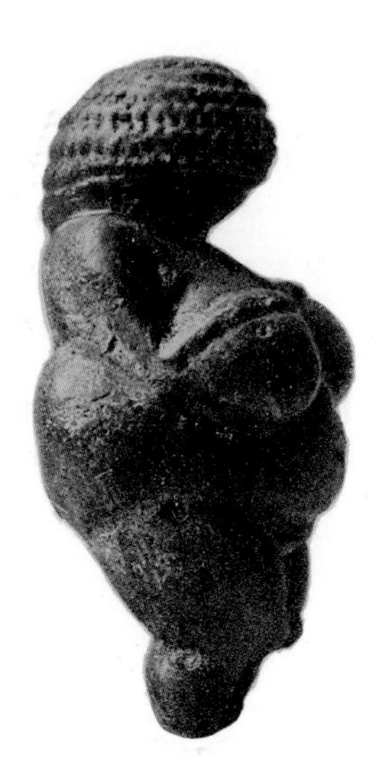

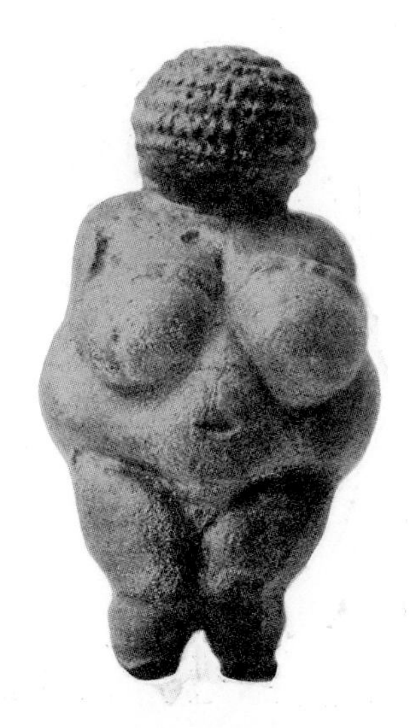

A female Paleolithic figurine discovered in Austria. Also known as the Venus of Willendorf. (Image courtesy of the Wellcome Trust.)

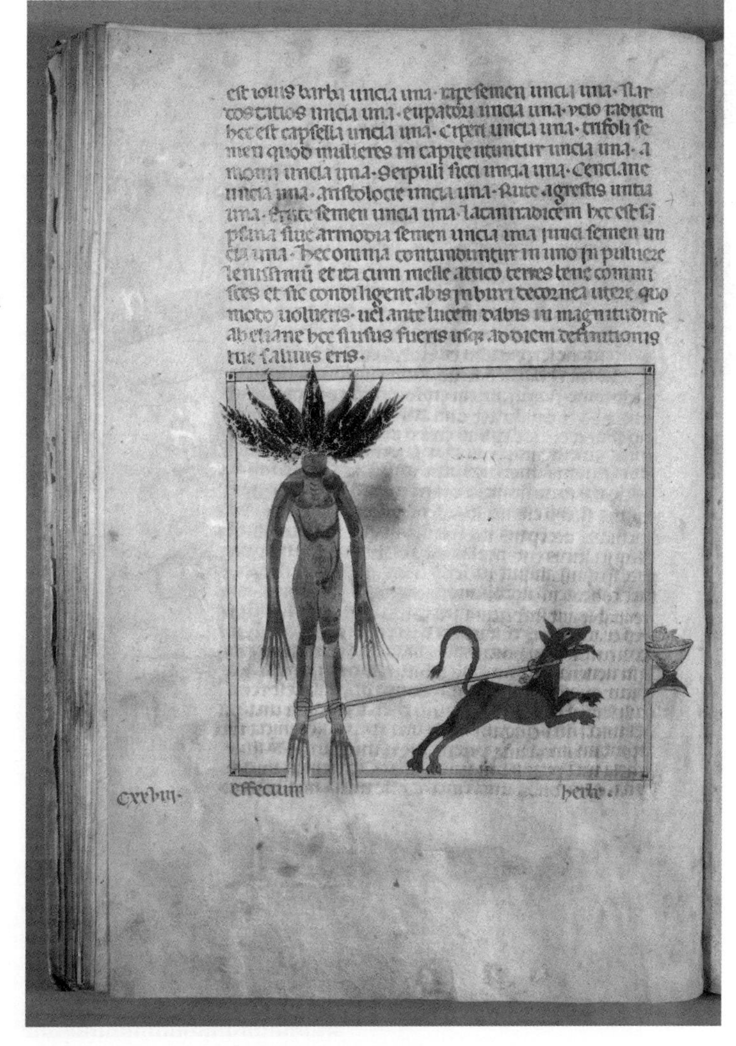

est iouis barba uncia una · rapesemen uncia una · sar
costicios uncia una · eupatori uncia una · pelo radicem
hec est capsella uncia una · cipen uncia una · trifoli se
men quod mulieres in capite utuntur uncia una · a
mom uncia una · serpuli sicci uncia una · Genciane
uncia una · aristolocie uncia una · Rute agrestis uncia
una · Eruce semen uncia una · lacian radicem hec est sa
psana siue armodia semen uncia una iunci semen un
cia una · hec omnia contunduntur in uno in puluere
lenissimũ et ita cum melle attico teres bene commi
sces et sic condiligent abis in bun decorrea utere quo
modo uolueris · uel ante lucem dabis in magnitudinē
abellane hec si usus fueris usq; ad diem definitionis
tue saluus eris ·

cxxviii· effectum herbe·

Mandrake being pulled up by a dog from the herbarium attributed to Pseudo-Apuleius. (Image courtesy of the Wellcome Trust.)

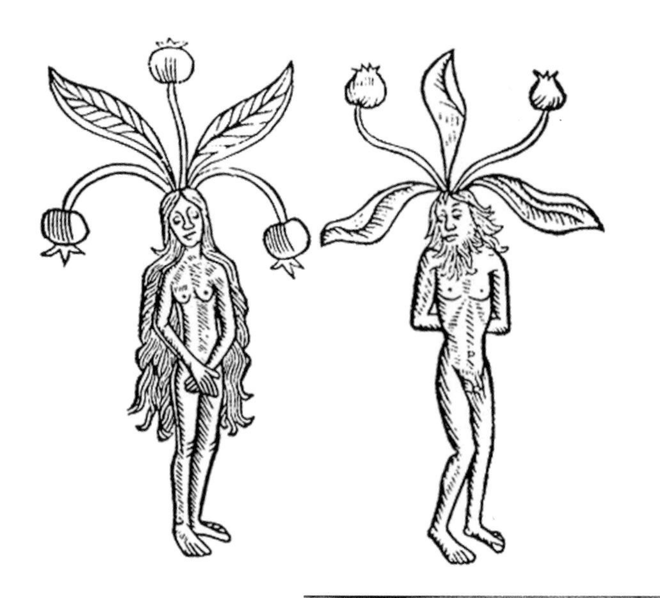

Representations of male and female mandrake roots from the fifteenth century *Hortus Sanitatis*.

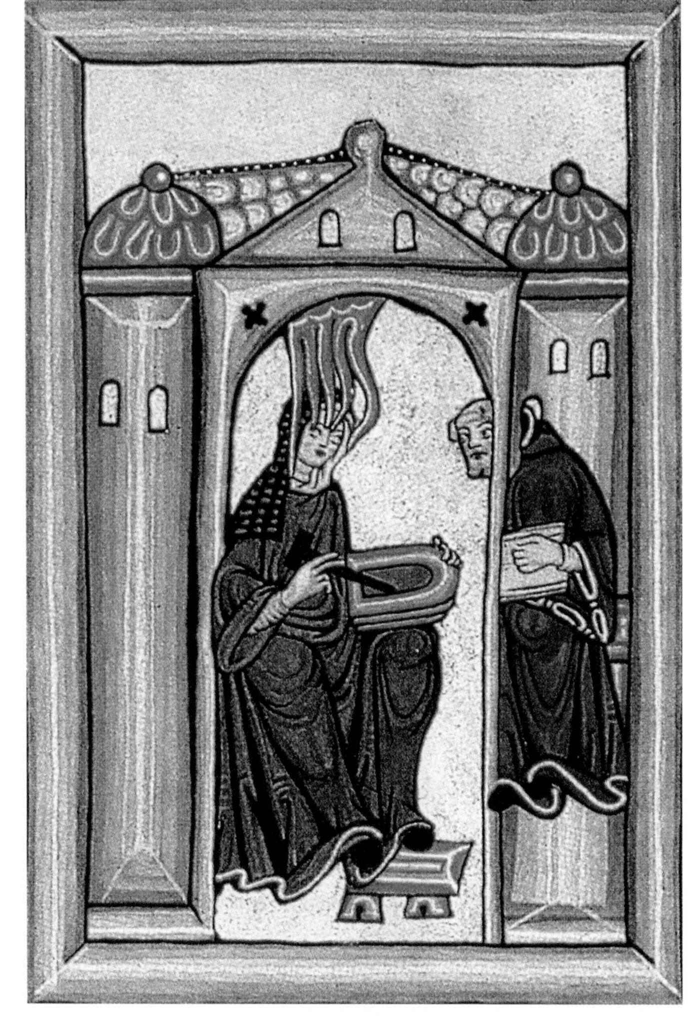

Saint Hildegard of Bingen using divination during one of her ecstasies.

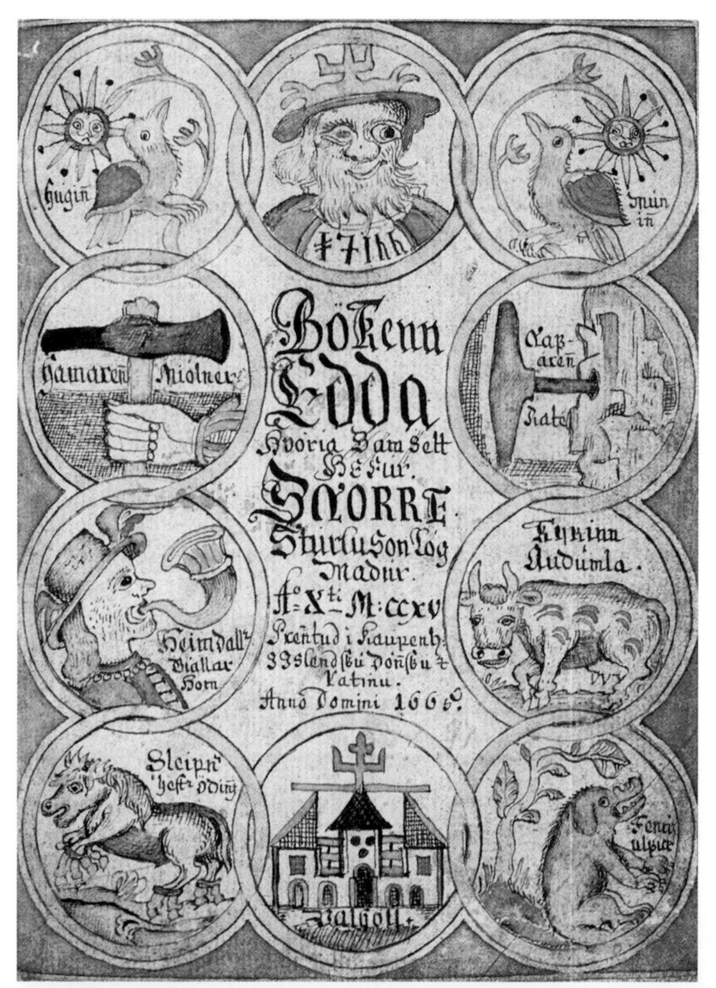

Illustration of the pagan god Woden (Odin) from the *Lacnunga* manuscript.

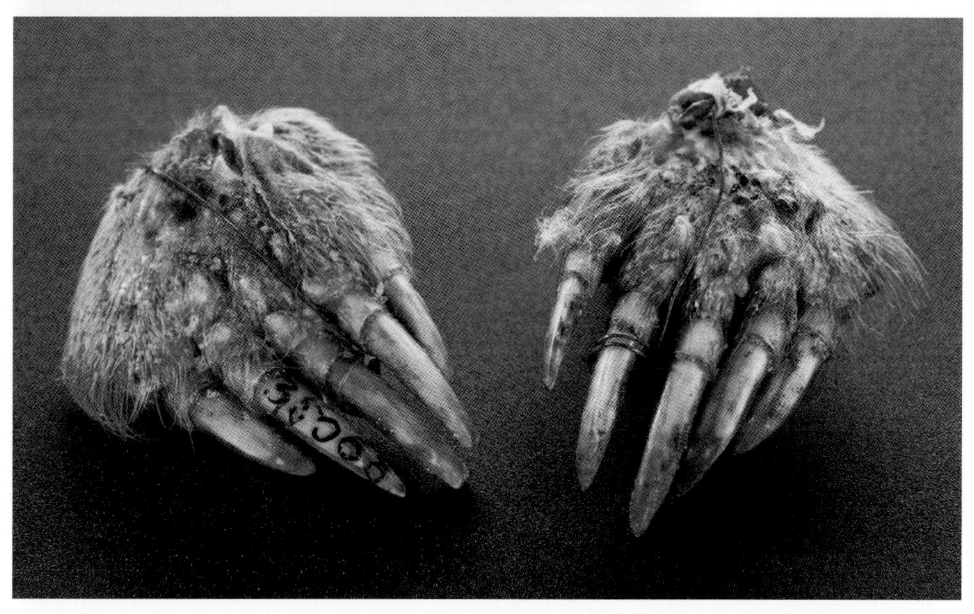

Mole's foot amulet from Norfolk, England. (Image courtesy of the Wellcome Trust.)

A rare example of a surviving twelfth century vellum leaf from Snorri Sturluson (1178-1241).

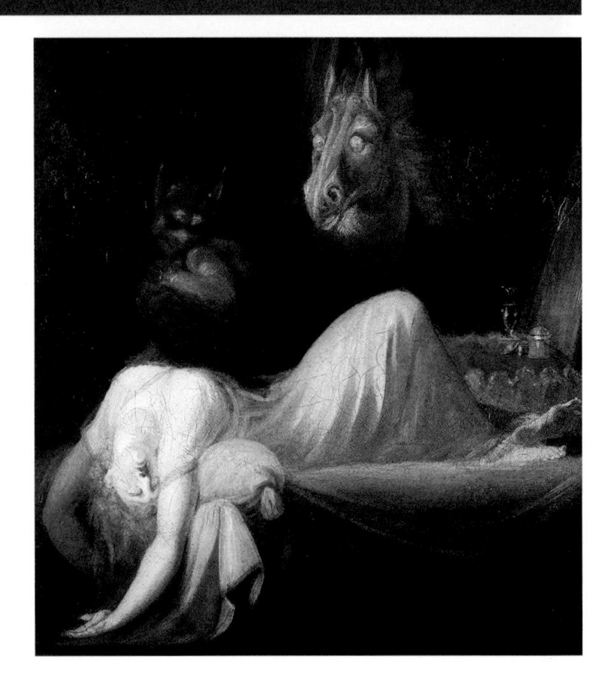

Fuseli's *The Nightmare*, 1790. Depicting a supernatural creature sitting upon the victim's chest.

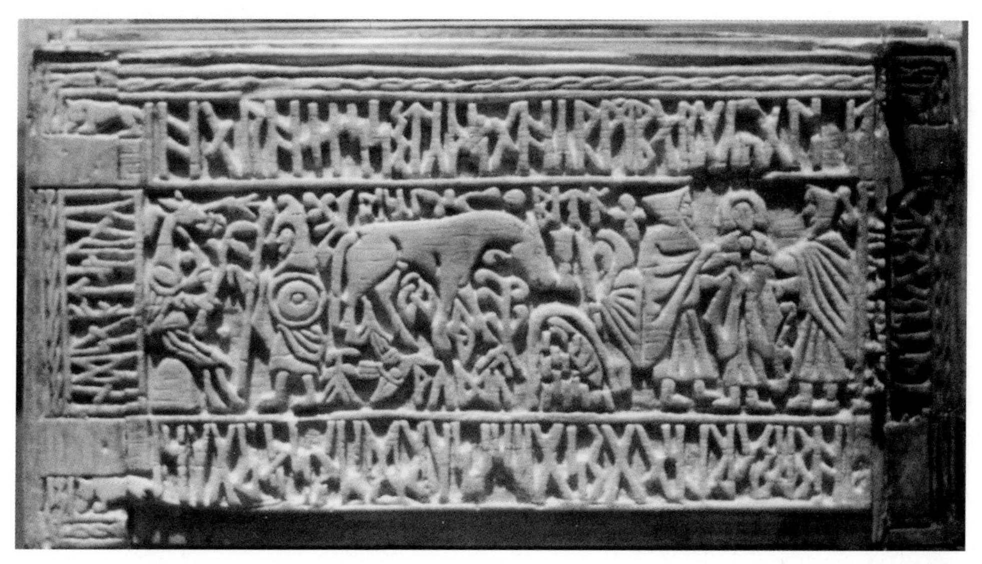

The Franks Casket, eighth century. The three Norns can be seen on the right. (Photograph by Mike Peel.)

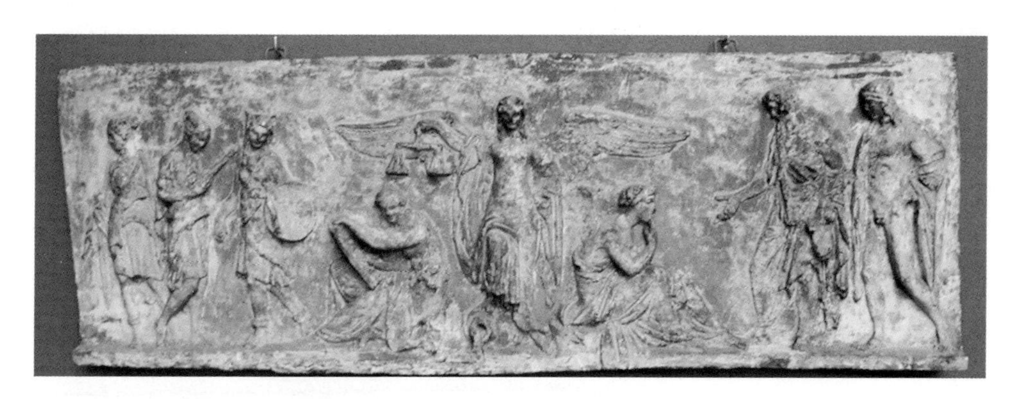

A photograph of *Mímir and Baldr Consulting the Norns* (1821-1822) by H.E. Freund, housed at the Ny Carlsberg Glyptotek, Copenhagen, Denmark.

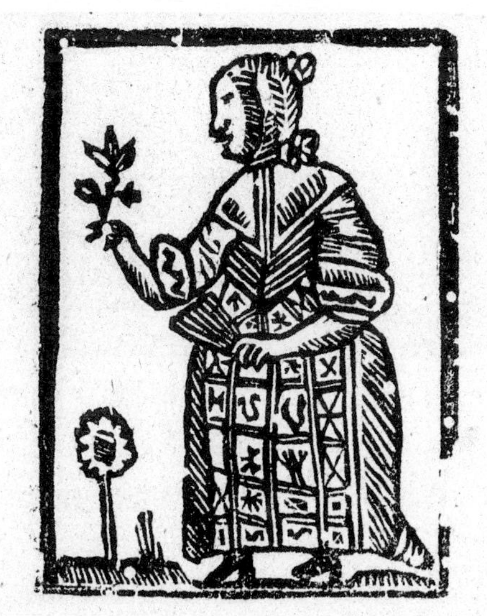

Woodblock illustration of a woman collecting herbs.

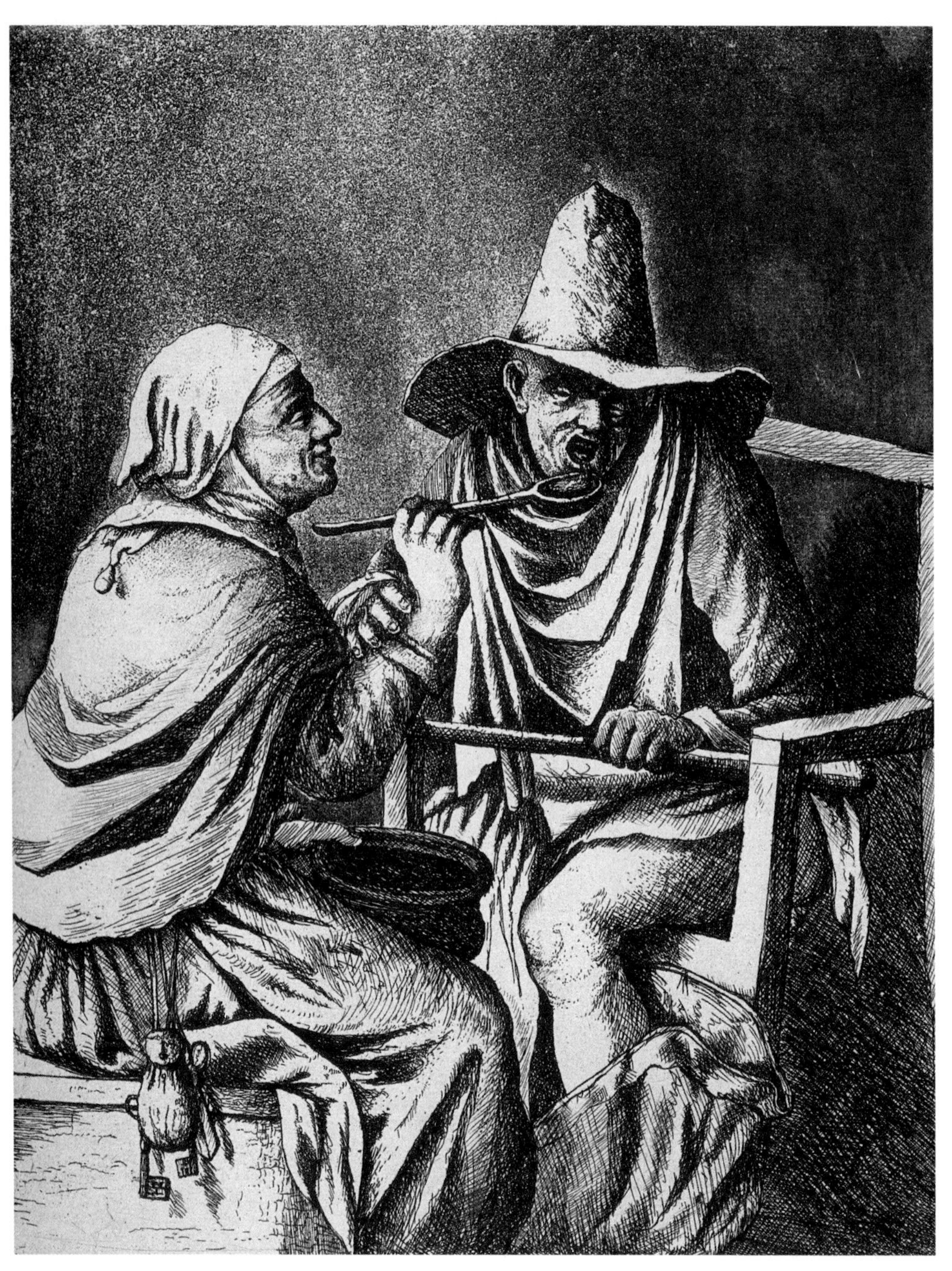

Illustration of an Anglo-Saxon folk-healer with her patient. An amulet hangs from her waist. (Image courtesy of the Wellcome Trust.)

or any from the west among the people.
Christ stood over diseases of every kind.

I alone know a running stream, and the nine adders beware of it.
May all the weeds spring up from their roots, the seas slip apart,
all salt water, when I this poison blow from you.

Mugwort, plantain open form the east, lamb's cress, venom-loather, camomile, nettle, crab-apple, chevil and fennel, old soap; pound the herbs to a powder, mix them with the soap and the juice of the apple.

Then prepare a paste of water and of ashes, take fennel, boil it with the paste and wash it with a beaten egg when you apply the salve, both before and after.

Sing this three times on each of the herbs before you prepare them, and likewise on the apple.
And sing the same charm into the mouth of the man and into both his ears, and on the wound, before you apply the salve.'

The nine-glory twigs are references to the runes (the ancient Germanic alphabet) brought back by Odin from his initiation while hanging upside-down upon the world tree. Odin hung upside-down for nine nights, where he died to the mortal world, travelled to the Otherworld, conversed with the dead and magical beings and then returned, reborn, with new knowledge.

Each runic letter is sacred to a specific herb. We learn from the story that singing the correct rune over a plant causes the herb to reveal its own otherworldly nature that has the power to thwart the worst poisons and diseases of this world. It is probable this singing and focused intention was also combined with visualisation as Paracelsus, writing in the early sixteenth century explains:

'He who is born in imagination finds out the latent forces of Nature, [and] He who imagines compels herbs to put forth their hidden nature.'

Although greatly respected within the medical establishment, Paracelsus retained a marked interest in the old ways of healing, which recognised that we live within an animated and interconnected reality. He was fascinated by alchemy and the occult, always pursuing the spiritual facet of medicine and healing whenever convention allowed. Paracelsus recognises ritual as awakening the higher imagination that would enable the initiate to behold the innate power of herbs.

The Nine Herbs Charm describes how the herbs battle with the forces of evil and this warring motif is frequently used in ritualistic remedies to situate the context of the healing. Trials and battles are similarly common devices used in initiations and it might be, if Bates is correct, that the power of plants aids the candidate through the psychological and physical aspects of the ceremony. The herbs thyme and fennel are being used in this charm to 'shape' the god Odin as he hung upside-down upon the world tree, experiencing his initiation. 'Shaping' implies a tutorial role with herbs acting as identities in their own right. Herbs therefore, are powerful enough to shape and teach a god.

It has been suggested that the herbs in the Nine Herbs Charm may also be the ingredients for a famous yet long lost concoction known as flying-potion. We know from the Norse Sagas and further Old Norse and Old English stories that flying-potion (also called flying-mead) was used in ancient initiation rites and shamanic ceremonies. Flying-potion may also have fuelled the witchcraft hysteria where the clergy declared that witches flew through the air and down chimneys. Flying-potion did not of course cause anyone to physically fly, but it may have been psychedelic enough to create a belief in flying. Those partaking of the flying-potion may have experienced such vivid, life-like adventures that they returned with an actual belief in their own ability to fly, or it could be that their stories of psychedelic trips became part of a common supernatural assumption.

Odin is specifically described as drinking this concoction to aid his shape-shifting abilities. Shape-shifting is equally as improbable as flying, yet with the herb mugwort, known for its psychedelic and hallucinatory effects (evidenced by the unregulated use of absinthe) this may well contribute to such experiences and the myths which then formed around them.

Mugwort and the other herbs do suggest an initiatory ordeal, specifically one relating to death and rebirth. Chamomile has qualities that would balance those of mugwort. It is a sedative and promotes the release of melatonin, so may negate some of the more anxiety-promoting aspects of mugwort, providing a more positive experience. Yet in large doses, chamomile can also be hallucinatory. Atterloathe is sometimes translated as black nightshade or deadly nightshade and other times as betony, so we will never know for sure what this herb actually is. We can say, however, that betony was used to ward off evil spirits and that black nightshade brought knowledge of death, which would be quite pertinent to a ritual requiring initiation through a symbolic rebirth. Thyme was also employed as a funerary plant as it was believed it helped the transition of the soul from this to the Otherworld. Fennel was often used to guard against evil whilst promoting immortality.

The Nine Herbs Charm would, as it directs, have been sung or chanted and as Malcolm Cameron states, it would have had a 'marvellously incantatory effect' upon the psyche, aiding an altered state of consciousness. The smiting of the snake also has great initiatory significance. Serpents, snakes and dragons have long been associated with hidden treasure both physical and spiritual. Alchemists and initiates believed this treasure to be wisdom and thus the snake/serpent must be battled and slain to reveal knowledge to the initiate.

If this were indeed an initiation, perhaps for a future healer or shaman, then it would have had a profound effect on the participant. Hearing the tale of Odin's own initiation whilst experiencing the psychotropic flying-mead would have created a powerful experience aimed at promoting a personal change – dying to the psychological and social norms in order to be resurrected and transformed. Joseph Campbell in *Myths to Live By* (1972) warns of the dangers of attempting such a process without proper instruction, as to do so can cause a complete schizophrenic break, where the personality is lost rather than transformed. Joan Halifax describes the healer's initiation quite elegantly:

> 'The healer's initiation – whether in a cave, on a mountain, atop a tree, or on the terrain of the psyche – embraces the experience of death, resurrection, and realisation of illumination. Variations on the fundamental theme of death and rebirth are found in all mythological traditions, and an encounter with death and release into rebirth are immutable dimensions of most personal religious experiences. The initiatory crisis of the healer must therefore be designated as a religious experience, one that has persisted since at least Paleolithic times and is probably as old as human consciousness, when the first feelings of awe and wonder were awakened in primates.'
>
> (Joan Halifax, *Shamanic Voices, a survey of visionary narratives*, 1992.)

As Halifax suggests, this type of initiation was meant to create a crisis through which the candidate must navigate to receive the boon of illumination. Crisis is dangerous and maybe even more so with the inclusion of hallucinogens, but ancient cultures often believed that healers were born with the strength and gifts required for the training. A dream, sign or personal idiosyncrasy would mark a person as significant and worthy of training and apprenticeship, and therefore, more likely to survive the ordeal of the Nine Herbs Charm.

Chapter 7

Herbal Remedies

Monasteries have provided us with the majority of herbal manuscripts that survive today. Saint Hildegard was not the only member of the Church to find these healing customs of interest. A similar work to Bald's *Leechbook* was commissioned in the eleventh century at St Augustine's monastery in Canterbury and although the herbal is thought to be a copy of an earlier fourth century text attributed to Psuedo-Apuleius, it is a remarkable book of remedies including elaborate indications for the use of mandrake as well as wonderfully detailed illustrations of anatomically correct male and female mandrake roots. The scanned manuscript is available to view on the Bodleian Library website.

What follows is a selection of healing remedies for common complaints direct from Bald's *Leechbook III* and a few from *Lacnunga* too. There are hundreds of cures but I hope I have selected some of the best. These are reproduced as informative only, and it is not recommended that the reader use or recreate them in any way, as many of the ingredients are known to be poisonous and deadly. Always, of course, seek out a modern medical professional if you are suffering from an illness of any kind. No quantities for the herbal ingredients are mentioned in the remedies; healers probably had an instinctive ability when prescribing ingredients, learned from years of observing and experimenting. Poisonous plants may, therefore, have been used in tiny quantities, a little like homeopathic treatments are used today, although this can only be speculative.

The remedies are presented in original Old English, followed by the Modern English translations. I make suggestions regarding their herbal efficacy by drawing on contemporary pharmacological research that has isolated the active properties of many herbs. Herbal remedies are popular today and, arguably, have never truly disappeared. High Street retailers recommend St John's Wort for depression, chamomile for anxiety and echinacea for immunity among many others; familiar ingredients from these old remedies that are being re-discovered today.

Ritualistic and psychological considerations come from my own background in psychology, psychotherapy and folklore. Where no exposition occurs, this is because the remedy is either quite straightforward, or its contents are similar enough to others to require little formal comment.

A general tonic to ward off all illness:

> *'Wið adle, nim þreo leaf gageles on gewylledre mealtre meolce, syle þry morhgenas drincan.'*

> 'Against sickness: take three leaves of gale in boiled sour milk; give it to him to drink for three mornings.'

This first remedy 'against sickness' indicates its use as a preventative tonic, rather like taking echinacea is today. I have used the accepted translation here but it is interesting to note the word '*syle*'. Commonly translated as 'to give,' a more accurate rendering of the word is 'to support'. Therefore, we can add certainty that this remedy is intended as a supportive tonic, perhaps stimulating the immune system. But would it work?

The plant used is gale, also known as English Bog Myrtle although it is not used in herbal medicine today as it can be extremely toxic. As an emmenagogue (a substance that stimulates menstrual flow), it can induce abortion, yet it has a long history of medicinal use in small quantities, even forming the basis of beer in Northern England and Scandinavia before the popularity of the hop. A 1996 study demonstrated gale to be an effective repellent against 'mosquitoes and other haematophagous pests of man and livestock'. It has also been used as a topical antiseptic and for intestinal worms, so using three leaves from the plant might have some general benefits against intestinal parasites without incurring toxicity. Gale is intensely fragrant and its repellent properties may have further informed the view that it protected one from illness.

To cure a rash:

'Wið oman, genim ane grene gyred ond læt sittan þone man on middan huses flore, ond bestric hine ymbutan ond cweð o þars et o uilia pars et pars inopia est, alfa et o, initium et finis.'

'Against a rash: take one green rod and have the man sit in the middle of the house's floor, and strike a circle around him and say: "Oh part, and O vile part, and the part is useless; alpha and omega, beginning and end."'

This remedy has a rather cobbled together feel about it. Tracing a circle about oneself is an aspect of Celtic magical technique yet this is followed by a Latin banishment. It is unlikely these parts were originally together and even less likely that either were used to remedy a rash. The scribes may have been confronted with a number of old and difficult to decipher snippets of remedies and rituals and did their best to combine them into a semblance of reason.

A salve for flying venom and sudden eruptions:

'Sealf wið fleogendum attre ond frspryngum, nim hamorwyrt handfulle ond mægeðan handfulle ond wegbrædan handfulle ond eadoccan moran, sece ða þe fleotan wille, þære ðeah læst, clænes huniges ane æscylle fulle, nim þonne clæne buteran, þrywa gemylte ðe þa sealfe midweorcean wile, singe man ane mæssan ofer ðam wyrtum ær man hy tosomne do ond þa sealfe wyrce.'

> 'A salve for flying venom and sudden eruptions. Take a handful of hammer wort and a handful of maythe and a handful of waybread and roots of water dock, seek those which will float, and one eggshell full of clean honey, then take clean butter, let him who will help to work up the salve melt it thrice: let one sing a mass over the worts, before they are put together and the salve is wrought up.'

'Flying venom' sounds rather fanciful and has led a number of researchers to consider whether this remedy might be the basis of Odin's famous flying mead from Snorri Sturluson's prose *Edda Skáldskaparmál*. Snorri was an Icelandic poet and historian of the twelfth century who saved many ancient stories and folk tales from the frozen North. The mead, we are told in Sturluson's poem, caused Odin to change his form into that of an eagle and fly away. There is even a version of the flying mead sold in Scandinavia today called Suttungr Brew, after the character that first stole the flying potion from dwarves in the saga; it contains honey, lingonberries, pine roots and heather.

The psychotropic Nine Herbs Charm provides a more compelling argument for the origins of the famous flying-mead as the above remedy simply does not have the herbal elements to justify it. Yet it does offer the solution for what the Anglo-Saxons commonly called flying venom. Chamomile and plantain (*maythe* and *waybread*) are soothing anti-inflammatories which when combined with clarified butter and honey would have made a useful skin ointment. Hammerwort (from the nettle family) provides clarity here as it has what at first appears to be a counter-acting effect to the previous herbs, causing skin irritation rather than soothing. This irritation, however, causes a numbing of the skin and so this salve would have soothed inflammation whilst providing a mild anaesthetic effect. It could be suggested therefore, that when the Anglo-Saxons spoke of using remedies for flying venom they were referring to a salve for the stings and bites of flying insects. The 'sudden eruptions' could be skin ulcers or boils from an infected bite. These might also benefit from a soothing ointment.

To cure a bleeding mouth:

> *'Wið þon þe mon blode wealle þurh his muð, genim betonican þreora trymessa gewæge ond cole gate meoloc þreo cuppan fulle, ond drice, þonne bið he sona hal.'*
>
> 'Against when blood pours through his mouth: take three tremisses' weight of betony and three cups full of cool goat's milk, and let him drink; then he will soon be healthy.'

Tremisses were the currency of Late Ancient Rome and continued to be used by the Anglo-Saxons following its fall. Betony or wood betony is the only herb used here, combined with goat's milk. Betony is a woodland plant common to England and has a long history of medicinal efficacy and folkloric stories that lend witness to its long-standing effectiveness as a healing herb. Margaret Grieve relays two ancient superstitions regarding betony in her *A Modern Herbal* (1972). Apparently, so it is told, if two snakes are caught in a circle of betony, they will fight to the death. Also, if a stag is wounded, it will search out betony, eat it and be cured.

The medicinal actions of the herb are extensive and varied. It is a useful general tonic and an Old Italian saying from *Stachys betonica* recommends that 'you should sell your coat and buy betony'. Regarding bleeding from the mouth John Gerarde has this to say:

> 'It stayeth bleeding at the nose and mouth, and helpeth those that spit blood, and is good for those that have a rupture and are bruised. The green herb bruised, or the juice, applied to any inward hurt, or outward wound in body or head will quickly heal and close it up. It will draw forth any broken bone or splinter, thorn or other thing gotten into the flesh, also healeth old sores or ulcers and boils.'
>
> (*Herball, Generall Historie of Plantes*, 1597.)

The remedy in question is not referring to just spitting blood. *Wealle* translates as something akin to a dam giving way and its contents pouring forth over the land, sudden and uncontrollable. It is likely therefore, that the condition being treated here is the rupture of an ulcer.

A remedy for asthma:

> *'Wið angcbreoste, wyll holenrinde on gate meolce ond sup wearm nyhstig.'*
>
> 'Against asthma: boil holly-bark in goat's milk and sip it warm, having fasted.'

Angcbreoste is literally 'narrow breast' and generally thought to indicate the type of constriction experienced with asthma. Holly is known to be a purgative and expectorant due to its toxicity yet the bark is less poisonous and has been used as a calmative in folkloric remedies. No research currently supports its efficacy, however, and it is unlikely to have had any success in treating asthma except for perhaps providing some calming effects.

A cure for fainting attacks:

> *'Wið ðone swiman, nim rudan ond salfian ond finul ond eorðfig, bettonican ond lilian, cnuca ealle þas wyrta tosomne, do on ænne þohchan, ofgeot mid wætere, grid swyðe, læt sigan ut on sum fæt, nim þone wætan ond wyrm, ond lafa þin heafod mid, do swa oft swa þa þearf sy.'*
>
> 'Against fainting: take rue and sage and fennel and ground ivy, betony and lily; pound all these herbs together; put into one bag; steep with water; rub well, let it drip out into a vat; take the liquid and warm it and rinse the head with it; do likewise as often as may be needful.'

A remedy for insomnia:

> *'Slæpdrænc, rædic, hymlic, wermod, belone, cnuca ealle þa wyrte, do in ealað, læt standan ane niht, drince ðonne.'*
>
> 'A sleeping drink: radish, hemlock, wormwood, henbane; pound all the plants; put them into ale; let it stand for one night; let him drink it then.'

Please do not feel curious about trying this remedy for insomnia. Radish is a good tonic, packed full of vitamins and minerals but hemlock, wormwood and henbane are all extremely dangerous. Hemlock is a sedative and henbane is known to cause hallucinations. Wormwood may be included to counteract the worse side-effects of the other two, but is itself toxic. It is probable that this remedy, in the correct quantities, may well have been successful at promoting unconsciousness.

To cure a fever:

> *'Wið gedrif, nim snægl ond afeorma hine ond nim þæt clæn fam, menge wið wifes meolc, syle þicgan, him bið sel.'*
>
> 'Against a fever: take a snail and first make from it clean foam and mix with a woman's milk; then drink it; he will soon be well.'

Slime-treatment has been known and used for centuries. In England, slime was extracted from both snails and slugs and used in topical applications for warts and similar skin conditions. The slime contains allantoin, which stimulates collagen production and further useful skin nutrients such as elastin, proteins, glycolic acid and lactic acid.

In Oxford's Pitt Rivers Museum, there is an old specimen jar containing a slug impaled on a thorn. The label on the jar instructs, 'Go out alone and find a large black slug. Secretly rub the underside on the warts and impale the slug on the thorn. As the slug dies the warts will go'. In other parts of the UK such as Berwickshire, Northumberland and Lancashire, the museum suggests that a snail replaces the slug:

> 'Take a black snail, rub the warts with it, and then suspend it upon a thorn; as the snail melts away, so will the warts. This must be done nine nights successively, at the end of which time the wart will completely disappear.'

The principle of transference is being used in these remedies to aid the healing properties of the slime as a cure for warts. The leechbook remedy is for fever, however, and directs that the slime be added to a drink containing a 'woman's milk'. Using snail slime internally is rather unusual and, beyond this remedy, there is little mention of the habit.

To cure sea-sickness:

> *'Wið wæterseocnysse genim þas wyrte pe man bulbiscillitici ond oðrum naman glædene nemneð ond gedryge hy syððan eal onbutan, genim þonne innewearde, seoð on wætere, ðonne hyt wearm sy seocnys beon ut atogen þærh migðan.'*

> 'For water-sickness take this plant which one calls bulbiscillitici [squill] and by another name gladden and dry it all outwardly afterwards, then take the inside, boil in water, when it is warm mix thereto also honey and vinegar, give three draughts full, very quickly will the sickness be drawn out through the urine.'

For toothache:

> *'Wiþ toþece ceow pipor gelome mid þem toþum. Him biþ sona sel. Eft, seoð beolenan moran on stangum ecede oþþe on wine, sete on þone saran toþ ond hwilum ceowe mid þy saran toþe,*

> *he bið hal. Gif þa teþ synd hole ceow boþenes moran mid ecede on þa healfe.*
>
> 'For toothache chew pepper often with the teeth. He will soon be well. Again, boil henbane's root in strong vinegar or wine, set it on the sore tooth, and let him chew it with the sore tooth sometimes, he will be better. If the tooth has a hole, chew bothen's root with vinegar on that side.'

The Old English word for toothache is *toþece*, and when we realise the character '*þ*' is pronounced as our modern 'th' then the similarity between the old and modern word is revealed. This remedy is actually a small collection of tooth related items.

First there is a prescription to chew pepper. Although pepper is not native to the British Isles, it was available in Anglo-Saxon England although the cost was prohibitive to most. Pepper was used throughout Southern Europe for abscesses and toothache as it provides a degree of numbing to a localised area.

The next recommendation for tooth pain could be seen as the poor man's version of the previous remedy. This time the plant is henbane root and the English seventeenth century botanist Culpepper says of it, 'to stop the toothache, apply to the aching side'. When used as an external poultice, henbane does have anaesthetic properties but it would not be wise to apply the plant internally, even within the mouth. Henbane is extremely poisonous.

The final remedy here is happily neither expensive nor toxic. *Bothen* is another name for rosemary and even today you will find rosemary oil recommended for toothache by many alternative medical practitioners. Not only can it help to numb the pain but it acts as an antiseptic to fight the infection too.

For a cough:

> *'Wiþ hwostan wyl marubian on wætre godne dæl, geswet hwon, sele drincan scenc ful. Eft, marubian swiðe wyl on hunige, do*

> *hwon buteran on, sele iii snæda oþþe iiii etan, on neaht nestig besup scenc fulne mid wearmes þæs ærran drences.'*

> 'For a cough, boil horehound in a lot of water, sweeten a little, give a cupful to drink. Again, boil horehound thoroughly in honey, put a little butter in, give three or four slices to eat having fasted overnight, sip a cupful of the previously mentioned drink warm with it.'

The herbalist John Gerarde (1545-1612) recommends horehound for coughs and colds and Culpepper states:

> 'It helpeth to expectorate tough phlegm from the chest, being taken with the roots of Irris or Orris … There is a syrup made of this plant which I would recommend as an excellent help to evacuate tough phlegm and cold rheum from the lungs of aged persons, especially those who are asthmatic and short winded.'

The plant continues to be used widely today for coughs and so it seems probable that this remedy would have had some beneficial effects.

A cure for lustfulness and unlustfulness:

> *'Gif mon sie to wræne wyl hindheoloþan on wiliscum ealað, drince on neaht nestig. Gif mon sie to unwræne wyl on meolce þa ilcan wyrt, þonne awrænst þu. Wyl on eowe meolce, eft, hindhioloþan, alexandrian, fornetes folm hatte wyrt. Þonne biþ hit swa him leofost bið.'*

> 'If one is too lustful boil water agrimony in foreign ale, let him drink it at night, fasting. If one is not lustful, boil the same plant in milk, then you make that person lustful. Boil in ewe's milk, again, water agrimony, horse parsley and the plant fornets hand, then it will be as if it is dearest to him.'

Here we find three curious remedies for lust and love all linked together. The first two use the same plant, water agrimony, to remedy excessive lust, and then again to increase lust. The only difference being that the former uses ale as the carrier where the latter uses milk. The third remedy again uses water agrimony but this time includes also horse parsley and fornets hand.

Pharmacologically, water agrimony contains nothing that might increase or decrease desire. The ale, if drunk in large enough quantities would probably be more successful at calming lustfulness. The plants in these remedies may instead be included by virtue of their sympathetic correspondences rather than any medicinal effects. Water agrimony, for example, grows in particularly damp places as does horse parsley which also contains thick mucilage. Fornet's hand is wild orchid, the bulb of which resembles the male testicle and Bierbaumer states in his book *Old Names New Growth* (2009) that the 'sperm-like, slimy quality of the extracts and the smell of sperm emanating from the testicle shaped bulb enhances the belief', the belief being that the bulb is good for attracting desire and love. The final line of remedy indicates that this is probably an ancient love spell.

For spleen pain:

'Wið miltan sare genim þas wyrte ðe man bryonia ond oþrum na- man hymele nemneð, syle þycgean gemang mete, þonne sceal þæt sar lipelice þurh þone micgþan forð gan; ðoes wyrt is to þam herigindlic þæt hy man wið gewune drenceas gemencgeað.'

'For pain of the spleen, take this plant which calls bryonia and by its other name hop, give it to eat in his food, then the pain must pass mildly out through the urine; this herb is so praiseworthy that it stands against men's foolishness.'

For burns:

> *'Wiþ bryne, gif mon sie mid fyre ane forbærned nim wudurofan ond lilian ond hleomoc, wyl on buteran ond smire mid. Gif mon sie mid wætan forbærned nime elmrinde ond lilian moran, wyl meolcum, smire mid þriwa on dæg. Wiþ sunbyrne, merwe ifig twigu wyl on butran, smire mid.'*

> 'For a burn, if one is burnt with fire alone take a dog rose, and lily, and speedwell, boil in butter and smear with it. If one is burnt with liquid, take elm bark, lily's root, boil in milk, smear with it three times a day. For sunburn, tender ivy shoots, boil in butter, smear with it.'

Butter is a common ingredient within the texts as it would have provided a good foundation for salves and here we find it mentioned twice in relation to burns. Using butter and similar substances on burns is a common folk-tradition but one that would have caused more problems than it solved.

Our human instinct is to protect wounded and burned skin from exterior infection and to soothe the pain. Butter seems a rational response, yet unfortunately it acts to contain the heat thereby making the situation worse. Writer and broadcaster Claudia Hammond says that for burns:

> 'Ancient Egyptian papyrus dating back to 1500BC describes the use of mud, excrement, frogs boiled in oil and fermented goat dung. Greeks from the 4th Century BC preferred rendered pig fat while the Romans used a mixture of honey and bran followed by cork and ashes.'

For the British to be using butter for burns is not therefore something to be criticised. In fact, the remedies also use lilies which are known to act to reduce the scarring associated with burns and the University of Maryland has found elm bark to be effective in treating burns and ulcerative skin abrasions too. The middle cure in this little triad of burn remedies is probably the most useful as it directs lilies to be boiled in milk rather than being applied in butter.

To protect against painful gums:

> *'Wið þæra gomena sare gyf hwa þysse wyrte wyrttruman þe man cri- sion ond oðrum naman clæfre nemneð mid him hafað ond on his swyran byrð, næfre him his goman ne deriað.*
>
> 'For pain of the gums, if anyone has with him the root of this plant which one calls crision and by another name clover and carries it on his neck, his gums will never hurt him.'

Here we see evidence that 'lucky' clover is an old belief. Medicinally, clover has many uses and it is possibly that its wide range of applications informed the 'lucky' superstition. The remedy recommends that the patient should carry the roots of the plant around their neck suggestive of an amulet. If the patient's belief in the auspicious properties of the plant is great enough, then such an amulet may well have nurtured some degree of placebo effect.

For a spider bite:

> *'Wiþ gongewifran bite nim heene æg, gnid on ealu hreaw ond sceapes tord niwe swa he nyte, sele him drincan godne scenc fulne'.*
>
> 'For a spider's bite take a hen's egg, crush it raw into ale and fresh sheep's dung, so that he (the patient) does not know, give him a good cupful to drink.'

This remedy often brings a smile to the face of those who read it as it seems to epitomise the difference between our modern sophisticated medicines and the ignorance of our ancestors; after all, we would never ingest sheep's dung today. It is little wonder that the directions ask the healer not to reveal to the patient what is in the drink. Pharmaceutically, there may be more to sheep's dung than meets the eye.

Sheep's dung is particularly rich in nitrogen and potassium, with the latter being the third most prevalent mineral in the human body, vital for many healing processes and bodily tasks. Today, potassium's healing properties have been determined for recovery from stomach cramping, stroke and hypoglycaemia, bone strength, brain function, muscular strength, anxiety and metabolism. As an electrolyte, it is helpful for the efficient transmission of energy between nerves, supporting muscle function. Potassium is also an anti-inflammatory. Nitrogen is used by the body for cellular repair and aids the process of proteins through the liver.

The health benefit of eggs is widely known. They are a good source of protein and the vitamin biotin that is used by the body for cellular healing and the strengthening of hair and nails. This remedy may therefore have had beneficial effects. There were risks though, as dung often contains parasites and intestinal worms.

The Anglo-Saxons were not the only people to use animal excrement within their remedies. In the Oxford-educated physician John French's *The Art of Distillation* (1651), we find the following remedy for epilepsy:

> 'Take the brains of a young man that hath died a violent death, together with the membranes, arteries, veins, nerves, all the pith of the back … bruise these in a stone mortar til they become a kind of pap … pour as much of the spirit of wine, as will cover it three or four fingers breadth, put into a large glass and allow it to digest … half a year in horse dung.'

Suddenly, the sheep's dung doesn't sound so bad.

Chapter 8

Dead Men's Graves

Archaeological evidence from Anglo-Saxon inhumations reveals the stark reality that death in childbirth was commonplace. Numerous graves contain pregnant women where the foetus is found in-utero, transverse or in rare examples, extruded. Extruded (post mortem extrusion) refers to what has commonly been termed coffin birth. This is where the mother has died during childbirth and as her body decomposes following burial, the build-up of gases due to putrefaction causes the foetus to be expelled through the vaginal opening. Forensic physician Sydney Smith (1955) speculated that this would happen between forty-eight to seventy-two hours following death. Childbirth was, therefore, an exceptionally dangerous activity for our ancestors. As Sayer and Dickinson explain:

> 'the biggest single cause of death for women was childbirth. Whether death took place as a result of mechanical malpresentation, infection or blood loss, the root cause was undeniable.'
>
> (*Reconsidering obstetric death and female fertility in Anglo-Saxon England*, 2013)

It is perhaps unsurprising that some of the most intricate, well documented and at times ritualistic remedies from the leechbooks concern fertility, childbirth and associated issues, although whether recommendations such as waving moles in the air served any truly beneficial purpose beyond the emblematic remains to be seen.

This small number of leechbook remedies specifically for what we would today term 'women's issues' feature all sorts of complaints from infertility to 'woman's madness'. The first cure is for a woman who has obviously been experiencing past difficulties achieving a successful pregnancy. It is wholly ritualistic and draws upon deeply significant life and death symbolism:

> *'Gif wif ne mæge bearn beran, se wifmann we hire cild afedan ne mæg, gange to gewitenes mannes birgenne ond stæppe þonne þriwa ofer þa byrgenne ond cweðe þonne þriwa þas word: "þis me to bote þære laþan lætbyrde, þis me to bote þære swæran swærtbyrde, þis me to bote þære laðan lambyrde" ond þonne þæt wif seo mid berane ond heo to hyre hlaforde on reste ga, þonne cweþe heo: "up ic gonge, ofer þe stæppe mid cwican cilde, nalæs mid cwellendum, mid fulborenum, nalæs mis fægan" ond þonne seo modor gefele þæt bearn si cwic, ga þonne to cyrican ond þonne heo toforan þan weofode cume cweþe þonne: "criste ic sæde þis acyþed."'*

> 'If a woman cannot bear a child, let the woman who cannot nourish her child go to the grave of a dead man and then step three times over the grave and say these words three times: "This is my remedy for hateful slow birth, this is my remedy for a difficult birth, this is my remedy for imperfect birth." And when the woman will be with child and goes to bed, to her husband, then she is to say: "Up I go, step over you, with a living child not a dying [one], with a full-born [one] not with a doomed [one]" and when the mother feels that the child is alive, she is to go then to a church and when she comes before the altar she is to then say: "To Christ I said, declared this."'

Ritualistic elements alone form this remedy; although it is most probable that it would once have been used in conjunction with herbs as part of a larger cure. The word *bote* is interesting. It generally means 'to get better,' but actually, its older meaning is more nuanced, implying a healing that occurs in response to an amends made. It is not unusual for people to believe that they have attracted ill fortune or disease into their lives due to some past aberrant action they have committed. Today we call this notion karma.

The ritual of stepping three times across the grave of a dead man and then again across her living husband is deeply symbolic. The woman is stepping across the boundaries of life and death with the number three symbolising completion and wholeness. L. Weston in *Women's Medicine, Women's Magic* (1995), agrees that the grave may be symbolic of a boundary between the living and the dead:

> 'The woman bearing a not-yet-living child embodies a similar boundary within herself.'

The ritualistic element extends into the words to be spoken. We find significant alliteration of *laþan lætbyrde* and *swæran swærtbyrde.* Such linguistic devices are common to invocations and chants and we can see how the patient is being specifically advised by the healer to recite words and act in certain ways. The finale of this remedy is to go to a church and declare these intentions to Christ.

To relieve womb and stomach pains:

> *'Wiþ wambewærce ond ryselwærce þær þu geseo tordwifel on eorþan up weorpan ymbfo hine mid twam handum mid his geweorpe, wafa mid þinum handum swiþe ond cweð þriwa: Remedium facio ad uentris dolorem. Weorp þonne oferbæc þone wifel on wge, beheald þæt þu ne locige æfter. Ðonne monnes wambewærce oððe rysle, ymbfoh mid þinum handum þa wambe, him bið sona sel, xii. Monaþ þu meaht swa don æfter þam wifele.'*

> 'For womb pain and stomach pain, where you see a dungbeetle on the ground casting it up, surround it with your two hands, with it upcast, wave vigorously with your hands and say thrice: "Remedium facio ad uentris dolorem" (A remedy suitable for womb pain), then throw the beetle away backwards, make sure

> that you do not look at it; then surround the person's womb or stomach pain with your hands, the womb will soon do better. You may do this for twelve months after the beetle.'

This remedy is clearly written down to give advice and direction to a healer. The healer is taught what to do over the course of the coming twelve months to relieve what may be persistent menstrual pains. The first thing to do is to locate a dungbeetle. Cockayne never believed that a dungbeetle was the original word within this cure however. He thought a later scribe either changed the ingredient or simply didn't understand the original term. Instead, he believed the ingredient was a mole.

Wayland Debs Hand has collected many folk beliefs concerning moles in his book *Magical Medicine: The Folkloric Component of Medicine* (1981), and describes several uses for the humble mole in Anglo-Saxon England. Moleskin would be wrapped around parts of the body to diminish cramps and muscle aches with bags of mole's feet carried upon the person to relieve rheumatic pain. The Anglo-Saxons had a particular tradition of waving moles around and imbuing their power for healing purposes and that, I would suggest, is what is happening here.

This remedy contains an ancient folk belief that moles have medicinal energy that may be harnessed by the healer. As late as the eighteenth century, Francis Grose in his 1790 work *A Provincial Glossary* describes the belief that if one holds a mole in the hand, squeezing it until it dies, that hand will acquire healing powers.

Why the Anglo-Saxons waved the mole about is unknown, but perhaps it was thought that waving it would loosen its energy to flow into the healer and by not looking at the mole, the healer could be sure the energy would not jump back to the creature. The description in the remedy that the beetle would be 'casting up' the ground lends further credence to Cockayne's instinct, as moles do indeed 'cast up' the earth. Why the scribe used dungbeetle instead, we may never know.

A remedy for morning sickness:

> *'Wið morgenwlætunga, wyl on wætre eorþgeallen, swet mid hunige, sele him godne bollan fulne on morgenne.'*
>
> 'Against morning sickness: boil earthnavel [knapweed] in water, sweeten with honey; give him [her] a good bowl full in the morning.'

Knapweed, a relation of the humble cornflower, was used readily as a general health tonic. Believed to aid digestion, stimulate appetite and cure ulcers, one can see a logical step in using it for morning sickness. Combined with honey, this would likely have been a reassuring, helpful drink.

A remedy for painful breasts:

> *'Wið breostwærce, marubie, nefte, ontre, bisceopwyrt, wenwyrt, wyl on hunige ond buteran, do þæs huniges twæde ond þære buteran þriddan dæl, nytta swa þe þearf sie.'*
>
> 'For breast pain, horehound, catmint, radish, bishopwort, wenwort, boil in honey and butter, put two thirds of honey to one third of butter, use it as it may be needful to you.'

Catmint has often been used as an anti-inflammatory for all manner of swellings. Culpepper recommends a salve of catnip for haemorrhoids stating, 'The green leaves bruised and made in to an ointment is effectual for piles'. Radishes are rich in nutrients such as vitamin C, zinc and phosphorus that are good for skin and scars and bishopswort is helpful for arthritic pain. Combining these herbs would certainly be of some relief for painful or swollen breasts. Wenwort is difficult to identify. It is commonly thought to be lesser celandine, although this is not definitive. Lesser celandine is actually caustic to the skin and causes, as Pliny describes:

'blisters like those caused by fire, hence the plant is used for the removal of leprous spots. They form an ingredient in all caustic preparations.'

Despite its caustic action, lesser celandine is included in many remedies for haemorrhoids. One might imagine how very painful this must have been, but given Pliny's advice that the plant helped to remove leprous spots, the caustic action may also have helped to sever the haemorrhoid from its attachment to the skin.

A further remedy for womb pain:

'Wiþ wambewærce ofgeot polleian ond drince ond sume binde to þam nafolan ond wite georne þæt sio wyrt aweg ne aglide; sona bið sel.'

'For womb pain, steep pennyroyal and let him [her] drink it, and bind some to his [her] navel, and be certain that the plant should not slip away; it will soon be better.'

We have seen pennyroyal used previously as a way of abortion. In small quantities, however, it was used and is used still, for menstrual cramping as it can have a soothing effect on the muscles and reduces pain. The plant is nonetheless toxic, and should not be used unless prescribed by a qualified clinical herbalist.

To induce menstruation:

'Wiþ þon þe wifum sie forstanden hira monaþ gecynd wyl on ealað hleomac ond twa curmeallan, sele drincan ond beþe þæt wif on hatum baþe ond drince þone drenc on þam baþe. Hafa þe ær geworht clam of beordræstan ond of grenre mucgwyrte ond merce ond of berene melwe, meng ealle tosomme, gehrer on pannan, clæm on þæt gecynde lim ond þone cwið nioþoweardne þonne hio of þam baðe gæp ond drince scenc

> *fulne þæs ilcan drenches wearmes ond bewreoh þæt wif wel ond læt beon swa beclæmed lange tide þæs dæges, do swa tuwa swa þriwa swæþer þu scyle; þu scealt simle þam wife bæþ wyrcean ond drenc sellan on þa ilcan tid þe hire sio gecynd æt wære, ahsa þæs æt þam wife. Gif wife to swiþe offlowe sio monað gecynd genim niwe horses tord, lege on hate gleda, læt reocan swiþe betweoh þa þeoh up under þæt hrægl þæt se mon swæte swiþe.'*
>
> 'For that their menstrual be absent from women, boil in ale speedwell and two centauries, give it to drink and bathe the woman in a hot bath, and let her drink the drink in the bath; have already made for yourself a poultice from beer dregs and from green mugwort and wild celery, and from barley meal, mix them all together, stir together in a pan, daub it onto the genital area and onto the lower part of the vagina, when she gets out of the bath, and let her drink a cupful of the same drink warm, and cover the woman well and let her be thus daubed for a long time in the day, do thus twice or thrice as you may have to; you must always make the bath and give the drink to the woman at the same time as would be normal for her [menstruation], ask this [time] of the woman. If the menstruals flow too strongly from a woman, take fresh horse droppings, lay it onto hot coals, let it smoke well between the thighs upwards under the clothing so that the person should sweat greatly.'

The absence of menstruation, known as amenorrhea, can have many causes such as malnutrition and thyroid or pituitary issues resulting in hormonal irregularities. The advice here is to brew together the herbs speedwell and centaury to produce a warm drink which should be given to the patient whilst in a hot bath. The timing is important. This must be done when the women would normally anticipate her period.

Centaury was used as a general tonic and for purifying the blood. Speedwell is an expectorant and continues to be used by herbalists today for coughs and colds. The poultice to be applied includes the emmenagogue mugwort mixed with wild celery, which is good for relieving anxiety. The action of mugwort may therefore have produced some allopathic results but the other ingredients suggest a particular understanding of the possible causes of the complaint from the perspective of the folk-healer.

Speedwell, centaury and celery are all calmative and combined with a warm bath and the relaxation that must necessarily occur to enable the consistent application of the poultice, I would suggest indicates that this remedy might be beneficial for the relief of anxiety and stress. Stress-induced amenorrhea is a recognised condition today and although little formal research on early psychology has been conducted, it could be suggested that this prescription fulfils the criteria of a psychological intervention.

For a woman's madness:

> *'Wiþ wifgemædlan geberge on neaht nestig rædices moran, þy dæge ne mæg þe se gemædla sceþþan.*
>
> 'For a woman's madness, let her eat radish's root at night having fasted, for that day the madness may not harm you.'

Radish is a mild antispasmodic and would have been useful for relieving menstrual pain. It could be, therefore, that what we term today 'women's issues', including PMS, was put rather less diplomatically twelve hundred years ago.

Chapter 9

Devils, Elves and Nightwalkers

To complain of devil-sickness today would probably result in a psychiatric referral. Old English remedies for devil-sickness, elf-sickness, nightwalkers and similar are generally understood to be extreme examples of psychological complaints that defied the understanding of our ancestors to such a degree that devils and their kind were the only reasonable explanation.

The diagnostic criteria for many psychological and neurological conditions did not begin until relatively recently. Schizophrenia was 'discovered' in 1887 for example and Alzheimer's in 1906. Further disorders then started to be extracted including psychosis, neurosis and psychopathy among others, providing us with a meticulously exhaustive system of psychiatric classifications. Although some distinctions were known within the classical world, emerging from Hippocrates' method of humours, researchers generally conclude that the unsophisticated Northern Europeans had no such discernment. In relation to epilepsy for example:

> 'The idea that epilepsy is a supernatural, demonic or spiritual disorder persisted with widespread beliefs that it was due to possession by the devil, a notion which obtained support from the miracle story of the cure of the epileptic child recorded in three Gospels. Epilepsy was also viewed as a result of a person perpetrating evil doings, or as a consequence of cycles of the moon or mystic magical phenomenon.'
>
> (Tempkin, *A Disease Once Sacred*, 1971)

Epilepsy is a neurological rather than psychological issue but if recent research by Peter Dendle of Pen State University is correct, then devil-sickness is not a catch-all psychological category from the barbarian past but rather, a sophisticated attempt by our ancestors at observing, experimenting and discerning, a remedy specific to epilepsy.

The key to unlocking Peter Dendle's theory that devil-sickness refers to epilepsy, is the plant lupin. Lupin is popular today and can be found flowering abundantly in many gardens throughout the summer in a variety of vibrant colours. Although its seeds have been used in cooking for centuries, Dendle found that when it came to devil-sickness remedies, lupin is always present:

> 'The most frequently prescribed herb for "devil-sickness" in the vernacular medical books from Anglo-Saxon England, the lupine, is exceptionally high in manganese. Since manganese depletion has been linked with recurring seizures in both clinical and experimental studies, it is possible that lupine administration responded to the particular pathophysiology of epilepsy. Lupine is not prescribed for seizures in classical Mediterranean medical sources, implying that the Northern European peoples (if not the Anglo-Saxons themselves) discovered whatever anticonvulsive properties the herb may exhibit.'

It is of course unlikely that the Anglo-Saxons knew specifically about manganese, yet through experimentation and observation they may have noticed that lupine acted to calm seizures. As lupin does not feature as an anti-convulsive in classical herbals, it is possible that this discovery was unique to the Old English folk-healers. Here is one of the curative drinks identified by Dendle from Bald's *Leechbook III*:

> '*Wiþ deofle, liþedrenc ond ungemynde: do on ealu cassuc, elehtran moran, finul, ontre, betonice, hindheolope, merce, rude, wermod, nefte, elene, ælfþone, wulfes comb; gesing xii mæssan ofer þam drence ond drince, him biþ sona sel.*

> 'For a devil and for madness, a mild drink: put into ale hassock, lupin's roots, fennel, radish, betony, hindhealth [water agrimony], marche, rue, wormwood, catmint, elecampane, elfthon, wolf's comb; sing twelve masses over the drink and let him drink it; it will soon be better for him.'

As Dendle contends, lupin is present as a main ingredient in this remedy for a devil and madness. I have noticed, however, that lupin is rarely used in isolation and other plants such as betony (bishopswort), fennel and radish are often found alongside it.

Hassock, a grass possibly similar to sedge, is the first plant mentioned here. Hassock and sedge feature in many remedies as restoratives and so this would have provided a good foundation for the remedy. Rue, betony and radish have their own anti-spasmodic and muscle relaxing virtues and may act complimentarily to lupin, enhancing its actions. Although wormwood does not appear to have any specifically antispasmodic actions, Gerarde states in his writings that our ancestors used wormwood and betony within remedies for 'falling sickness' or epilepsy.

The inclusion of catmint, agrimony and fennel would have made this drink very pleasant to the taste, although Margaret Grieve considers fennel may have had significance beyond taste alone. She states in her *A Modern Herbal* that:

> 'In mediaeval times, Fennel was employed, together with St. John's Wort and other herbs, as a preventative of witchcraft and other evil influences, being hung over doors on Midsummer's Eve to warn off evil spirits.'

Fennel may thus serve a dual purpose in this remedy. As a talisman against evil it would augment the ritualistic recommendations of singing masses above the drink. As a medium for delivering a pleasant taste it could have ensured that a patient was able to take the remedy regularly. Although a one-off hit of foul tasting medicine can be tolerated, something that required daily use could prove too unpalatable without fennel.

Dendle's thesis relies, however, upon the manganese (not to be confused with magnesium) content of lupin. He correctly asserts that recent research has found a correlation between manganese deficiency and seizures, but it might also be possible that the magnesium rather than manganese content of lupin is equally beneficial for seizures. Dr Mark Sircus reports in *Transdermal Magnesium Therapy* (2007) that in a trial testing the effects of 450mg of magnesium taken daily by thirty epileptics, magnesium was successful in controlling seizures. A further study corroborated this research, demonstrating that seizures were most severe in patients with low levels of magnesium. Lupin has high concentrations of both magnesium and manganese and so would have been successful in the correct doses against the seizures experienced in epilepsy. It seems that Dendle's hypothesis may well be correct. Here is a further remedy, this time for the *deofles costunga* (devil's tempations):

> *'Drenc wiþ deofles costunga: þefan þorn, cropleac, eletre, ontre, bisceopwyrt, finul, cassuc, betonice, gehalga þas wyrta, do on ealu halig wæter, ond sie se drenc þærinne þær se seoca man sie, ond simle ær þon þe he drince, sing þriwa ofer þam drence: dues in nomine tuo saluum me fac.'*

> 'A drink for the devil's temptations: hawthorn, cropleek, lupin, radish, bishopwort, fennel, hassock, betony; hallow these plants, put holy water into ale and let the drink be inside where the sick person is, and always before he may drink it, sing thrice over the drink "dues in nomine tuo me fac".'

Lupin, hassock, fennel, betony and radish are all together again in this second remedy for a devil. The protective elements are equally recognisable. The Latin translates as 'God, save me in thy name' and is from psalm 53. We find similar ingredients in next remedy for devil-sickness indicating that a definite pattern is emerging:

> *'Wiþ deofolseoce do on halig wætre ond on eala bisceopwyrte, hindhioloþan, agrimonian, Alexandrian, gyþrifan, sele him*

drincan. Eft, cassuc, þefan þorn, stancrop, elehtre, finul, eoforþrote, cropleac, ofgeot gelice. Eft spiwedrenc wið deofle, nim micle hand fulle secges ond glædenan, do on pannan, geot micelne bollan fulne ealaþ on, bewyl healf, gegnid xx lybcorna, do on þæt. Ðis is god drenc wiþ deofle.'

'For devil-sickness, put into holy water and into ale bishopswort, hindhealth, agrimony, horse-parsley, cockle, give it to him to drink. Again, hassock, hawthorn, stonecrop, lupin, fennel, boarthroat, cropleek, pour out likewise. Again, a powerful drink for a devil, take a large handful of sedge, and of gladdon, put it into a pan, pour over a large bowl of ale, boil half away, crush twenty libcorns and add them to it. This is a good drink for a devil.'

There are in fact three remedies here, put together with the linking device 'again' used to bring literary coherence. Lupin, hassock, sedge, fennel and betony are all here although only the middle cure contains lupin and fennel. Betony is found in the first remedy and it might be that this cure is earlier, coming from a time before lupin was introduced to England in the seventh century. The final remedy is very different to what Dendle has described, however, and although sedge and gladdon would probably be included here as a general tonic, the libcorns demonstrate a very different approach to devils.

Libcorn has been translated as wild saffron, yet it is more likely to be meadow saffron, which was common to British woodlands. It is highly toxic but in the correct dosage is an effective emetic causing vomiting. Purging is not uncommon to the more supernatural remedies as the act was believed to rid the body of illness. As the monasteries increasingly controlled community healthcare, purging became popular due to the Christian belief that Satan caused disease and needed to be exorcised.

These three cures for a devil may therefore illustrate an evolution in how our ancestors treated epilepsy. We have herbal concoctions to relieve symptoms; first betony, which is a mild anti-spasmodic common to England, followed in the next cure by lupin, the more powerful foreigner. Lastly there is the supernatural response of purging, as seizures were increasingly thought to be the work of the devil within the Christian cosmology. This possible evolution of treatments from indigenous betony to the later lupin concluding in the Christian purging raises the question - Is lupin alone a reliable method of discerning cures for epilepsy?

In *Elf Charms in Context* (1996), Jolly suggests that charms for devil-sickness are in fact Christianised versions of earlier elf cures. If this is true then Dendle's hypothesis, that devil-sickness is a cure for epilepsy, should hold true for elf remedies also. To assess whether this is correct is problematic, however, as Dendle's methodology of using lupin as a standard of assessment does not work with elves as the plant wasn't present in Britain until the seventh century.

We therefore have a dual problem; lupin appeared on the scene as a newcomer, just as pagan elves were transforming into Christian devils. Yet, if Jolly is correct, I would expect to find two things occurring in the manuscripts. Firstly, I would look for transitional aspects in the remedies. For example, there should be some elf-sickness cures that do contain lupin and equally, some devil-sickness charms that do not. Secondly, I would look for the plant common to the earlier elf remedies that may show some anti-convulsive properties, as this plant could be a pre-cursor to the later more powerful lupin. A charm against elf-sickness from a previous chapter states:

> 'For elf-sickness, take bishopwort (betony), fennel, lupin, the lower part of elfthon, lichen from the hallowed sign of Christ, and storax, take a handful of each, bind up all the plants in a cloth, dip it into hallowed font water thrice …'

The remedy then continued, directing the healer to smoke the patient and provide a tonic. This elf-sickness remedy contains the ingredients we have come to expect from devil-sickness. Bishopswort (betony), fennel, lupin and cleansing are all apparent here. Interestingly, betony is listed before lupin and it might be possible that betony was used before the introduction of lupin and here, at least, still takes centre stage. Many elf remedies contain similar ingredients, so it is possible that they were the forerunners of devil-sickness.

Within the texts, however, we find further remedies containing the same ingredients, but without the words devil or elf. Instead we find the more ambiguous designation of 'fiend'. Could fiend remedies also play a part in the discussion regarding epilepsy cures or is it just a coincidence that the herbs are the same? Today we generally think of the devil as being a fiend although this may not be true for our ancestors. Here is one such remedy:

> *'Wyre gode sealfe wiþ feondes costunga, bisceopwyrt, elehtre, haransprecel, streawberian wise, sio clufihte wenwyrt, eorðrima, brembel æppel, polleian, wermod, singe viiii mæssan ofer, smire þone man mid on þa þunwonge ond bufan þam eagum ond ufan þæt heafod ond þa breost ond under þam earmum þa sidan. Ðæs sealf is god wiþ ælcre feondes costunga ond ælsidenne ond lenctenadle.*

> 'Work a good salve for a fiend's temptations, bishopswort (betony), lupin, harespeckle, strawberry stalk, the cloved wenwort, earthrim, bramble fruit, pennyroyal, wormwood, pound the plants, boil them in good butter, wring through a cloth, set it under the alter, sing nine masses over it, smear the man with it on the temple, and above the eyes, and on top of the head, and the chest, and on the sides under the arms. This salve is good for all the enemy's temptations, and elf-bonds, and spring fever.'

This remedy for a fiend's temptations states at the end that it is good for three issues – the enemy's temptations, elf-bonds and spring fever. It seems unlikely that all three issues stated here relate to epilepsy, yet a fiend or enemy's temptations and the inclusion of herbs lupin and betony raise an interesting question – can we include this remedy as a cure against epilepsy or not? If we can then the boundaries of Dendle's idea are wider than he has so far considered.

Beginning with 'spring fever', Peter Clemoes writing in the twelfth volume of *Anglo-Saxon England* (1986) argues that it is a form of benign tertian malaria that swept the country following winter. British bioarcheological research does not support this theory, however, although the marshland of Anglo-Saxon England would certainly have been a ripe environment for malaria. It seems some type of feverish illness did exist, Chaucer and Shakespeare even mention it in their works, but it was not a form of malaria.

The next issue mentioned in the remedy for a fiend's temptations is 'elf-bonds' and Stephen Pollington suggests elf-bonds may mean 'enchanted by an elf' perhaps describing a kind of delirium. The purgative drink, he comments, could be part of an exorcism to drive out the evil spirit.

Within Bald's book three there are a number of remedies for being bound by bewitchment or enchantment:

> *'Gyf hwa on þære untrumnysse sy þæt he sy cis, þonne meaht ðu hine unbindan; genim þysse wyrte þe we leonfot nemdon fif ðyfelas butan wyrttruman, seoð on wætere on wanwægendum monan ond ðweah hine þærmid ond læd ut of þam huse on foran nihte ond ster hyne þære wyrte þe man aristolochiam nemneð ond þonne he utga ne beseo he hyne nu on bæc; þus ðu hine meaht of þære untrumnysse unbindan.'*
>
> 'If someone be in the affliction that he be "bewitched" you can unbind him then; take five bushes of this plant which we named lionfoot, boil in water under a waning moon and wash him with it and lead him out of the house before nightfall and waft him with the plant which is called smearwort and when he goes out let him not look back, thus you can unbind him from the affliction.'

Lionfoot is the common English name for Lady's Mantle (*Alchemilla Vulgaris*). Old herbals mention its 'binding' nature for wounds, and it was often used as a poultice, so symbolically; this plant may be sympathetically linked to the notion of supernatural bondage. A waning moon has the quality of diminishment and so to boil lionfoot during a waning moon would lessen the bewitchment.

Smearwort was a much-loved herb of Anglo-Saxon England. Although many modern herbals claim that smearwort did not and does not exist in England, it is clear from the Old English documents that it did and still does today. Confusion might have arisen due to the plant's alternative names, the most popular of which being Good King Henry. In Sauer's 1776 herbal, it states, 'Good King Henry … may be laid green on all angry rotten injuries'. Smearwort's many and varied medicinal virtues, from wound healer to digestive also attracted the name 'All Good'. It is not a stretch to consider that symbolically, smearwort may have been viewed as a lucky and protective amulet against the agendas of devils and elves.

The direction to 'not look back' is common in banishment rituals. The eyes have always been considered as routes to the soul and there is a tradition that one should never look evil in the eye as it may enter through such a gaze. But what did it mean to be bewitched? For there to be a remedy, bewitchment would suggest that our ancestors considered this to be an affliction and as Clive Holmes writes:

> 'the witch possession identification might prove seductive to those symptoms that bewildered medical experts, their families and neighbours and most crucially themselves.'
>
> (Clive Holmes, *Popular Culture, Witches, Magistrates and Divines in Early Modern England*, 1984).

I have used the accepted translation of *untrumnysse* as 'bewitched'. Yet *untrumnysse* is an early West Saxon word meaning a binding illness, not a witch, and *unbindan* literally means to unbind. So, an accurate translation of the first sentence is rather more like this: 'If someone is ill bound, see that he is careful, then you will be able to unbind him'. The assumption in translation that this refers to being bewitched is fair, however, as the Old English belief that an illness has been bound to a patient implies the action of sorcery. Bewitchment or elf-bonds may therefore have been a response to illness that left our ancestors 'bewildered' enough to ascribe sorcery as the only explanation.

Can we say the remedy for a fiend's temptations fits the category of devil-sickness and elf-sickness, thus broadening Dendle's classifications? With the inclusion of lupin and betony (bishopswort) and mention of a 'fiend', it seems likely. The inclusion of spring fever could be viewed as a secondary illness, also thought to have been sent by such creatures demonstrating an adaptability to this class of epileptic remedy.

Curiously, however, there is a methodological difference in the fiend remedy that does not fit with devil or elf-sickness cures and renders it useless for the treatment of epilepsy. In the devil and elf remedies, the concoctions are to be turned into a drink, to be ingested by the patient. This internal prescription, as we have seen, would be useful for calming seizures. In the remedy for a fiend's temptations there is no internal prescription. Rather, the herbs are to be turned into a salve so the healer should, 'smear the man with it on the temple, and above the eyes, and on top of the head, and the chest, and on the sides under the arms'. The action of smearing around the head and arms would have had no effect on epilepsy so it is probable that lupin and betony are being used here for a different purpose. If so, then we are now leaving Dendle behind and venturing into somewhat darker unventured territory where lupin and betony fight against an altogether more sinister creature – a nightwalker:

> *'Wyrc sealfle wið nihtgengan, wyl on buteran elehtran, hegerifa, bisceopwyrt, reade maðgan, cropleac, sealt, smire mid, him bið sona sel.'*
>
> 'Make a salve against nightwalkers: boil in butter lupin, hedgerive, bishopwort (betony), red maythe, cropleek, salt; smear with it, it will soon be better for him.'

This is very similar to the 'fiend' remedy and sheds light on a whole new ancestral world where people felt compelled to protect themselves against the *nihtgengan*. But what were 'nightwalkers' and what ailment did our ancestors believe they inflicted? Lupin and betony are certainly used here but as they are being turned into a salve rather than a drink, their pharmaceutical properties would likely be of little benefit. With little internal efficacy possible from such an ointment, we must look to other explanations such as folklore instead. For example, Margaret Grieve says of betony:

> 'In addition to its medicinal virtues, Betony was endowed with power against evil spirits. On this account, it was carefully planted in churchyards and hung about the neck as an amulet or charm, sanctifying, as Erasmus tells us, 'those that carried it about them,' and being also 'good against fearful visions' and an efficacious means of "driving away devils and despair". An old writer, Apelius, says: "It is good whether for the man's soul or for his body; it shields him against visions and dreams, and the wort is very wholesome, and thus thou shalt gather it, in the month of August without the use of iron; and when thou hast gathered it, shake the mould till nought of it cleave thereon, and then dry it in the shade very thoroughly, and with its root altogether reduce it to dust: then use it and take of it when thou needst."'

Betony has long been used as a device to ward off evil and may be included in the nightwalker remedy for amuletic purposes alone. The locus of intent for such a cure may thus be protection. Unlike the treatments identified by Dendle that aimed to cure an existing ailment, these nightwalker and fiend remedies seem clear in their focus of warding off some perceived future malady. Methodologically, this puts devil-sickness and nightwalker remedies in very different categories of therapy, one being curative and the other preventative. Grieve also mentions betony in relation to 'dreams', adding to the nocturnal element indicated by nightwalkers. We therefore have a treatment here for something that our ancestors perceived as attacking at night.

The first potential ailment builds upon this perception of nocturnal threat. The very word nightwalker is uncomfortable. It alludes to something that walks around at night whilst most ordinary folk are asleep in their beds and the whole character evokes an oppressive anxiety. Research recently conducted by the Southwest University in China has confirmed that humans have an evolutionary pre-disposition to be scared of the night. Their findings reported in the *International Journal of Psychophysiology* conclude that 'individuals are highly reactive to cues that signal potential threatening events at night.' For our ancestors, this evolutionary alertness for things that go bump in the night may have had greater significance than our current predisposition. Nightwalkers may thus refer to a primal experience of fear and anxiety surrounding the night.

The problem with this explanation is, however, that other nightwalker remedies make more specific mentions of evil, elves, temptation and succubae (nocturnal sexual spirits) implying along with the sheer quantity of such remedies, that something more formidable is going on. Anxiety may certainly be involved but it is unlikely to stand alone.

A further potential explanation for nightwalkers which is worth exploring comes from their similarity to the myth of vampires, a connection more easily discernable from the following more elaborate cure found in Bald's *Leechbook III*:

> *'Wyrc sealfe wiþ ælfcynne ond nihtgengan ond þam mannum þe deofol mid hæmð, genim eowohumelan, wermod, bisceopwyrt, elehtre, æscþrote, beolone, harewyrt, haransprecel, hæþbergean wisan, cropleac, garleac, hegerifan corn, gyþrife, finul, do þas wyrta on an fæt, sete under weofod, sing ofer nyan mæssan awyl on buteran ond on sceapes smerwe, do haliges sealtes fela on, aseoh þurh clað, weorp þa wyrta on yrnende wæter. Gif men hwilc yfel costung weorþe oþþe ælf oþþe nihtgengan, smire his ond wlitan mid þisse sealfe ond on his eagan do, ond þær him se lichoma sar sie, ond recelsa hine ond sena gelome, his þing biþ sona selre.'*

> 'Work a salve for elf-kind, and nightwalkers, and the people who have sex with the devil, take ewehumble, wormwood, bishopswort, lupin, ashthroat, henbane, harewort, whortleberry shoots, cropleek, garlic, hedgerive, corn cockle, fennel, put these plants into a vessel, set it under an alter, sing nine masses over it, boil in butter and in sheep's grease, add a lot of holy salt, strain through a cloth, throw the plants into running water. If any evil temptation should befall one, or an elf, or a nightwalker, let him smear his face with this salve, and put it on his eyes, and where his body may be sore, and smoke him, and make the sign over him often, his case will soon be better.'

All manner of nasties are mentioned in this cure. Nightwalkers, elves and unusually 'people who have sex with the devil'; this odd statement of affliction refers to succubae. Succubae were thought to be evil spirits that copulated with people at night whilst sucking their life force or soul from them during sleep. Lupin and betony feature again with a salve to be smeared on the face and eyes. Unravelling the mystery of such a remedy requires careful consideration of the ritualistic aspects and remaining herbal ingredients to ensure nothing is missed. To this end, I am grateful that the professional herbalist Susan Tosni offered her expert opinion regarding the latter.

Susan Tosni immediately noted the unusual ritualistic aspect of this remedy, something that is certainly uncommon within modern herbalism. Susan found that the herbs indicated were not always easily recognisable due to the varied way in which common plants names have been ascribed over the years. Therefore, when a number of alternatives are possible, she considered each one, arriving at the conclusion that with regard to the herbal ingredients of this cure, there are two main active principles elicited – firstly there are those which act to soothe and protect the skin and secondly, those with properties that would promote sleep and relaxation. Below is her herbal exposition:

> 'Ewehumble, Hops (*Humulus lupulus*) – Pollington gives Hops or Bryony as alternatives for this plant, although Shirley Kinney

assumes *eowohumelan* to indicate hops. The plant is typically used for its sedative, relaxing and hypnotic actions. Hop pillows are popular for promoting sleep and comforting mental strain. It is also used in anorexia because it promotes digestive action with its bitter content, the bitter flavour in beers, but the plant would have to be taken internally to have this action. It calms abnormal sexual excitability in both sexes and would be useful in priapism or premature ejaculation. There are reports of its application externally for painful swellings and boils having bacteriostatic and analgesic actions. The scent of the plant contributes to this.

If Pollington is correct and *eowohumelan* is bryony then this plant also has a sedative affect on the nervous system, controls temperature in fever and increases T cell activity and is therefore anti-infectious. It has a particular action as a pulmonary agent and has been used in acute infections including tuberculosis. It is used internally but the dose is restricted and therefore requires care. Externally it has a use as a rubefacient.

'Bishopswort – This may be one of several plants, betony, marshmallow, soapwort or verbena. Ashwort, however may be verbena. Betony (*Stachys betonica/ Stachys officinalis/Betonica officinalis*) has always been held in high esteem and is used today as a mild sedative and vulnerary with anti-venom capability. It has a particular affinity for the head and would be considered for a tension headache or facial neuralgia. As a sedative, it would be useful to calm someone in hysteria. These actions might be milder if the herb extract were applied to the skin. Its alternatives of Soapwort (*Saponaria officinalis*) and Marshmallow (*Althaea officinalis*) both have emollient properties useful for skin lotions for eczema, psoriasis and acne and the soothing and disinfecting of inflamed or irritable skin.

'Lupin (*Lupulus spp*) – This plant is rarely used today but the extracts of the seeds have been used on the skin as an emollient and to draw abscesses. Lupin features often in charms for elves and demons. The directions in this charm are topical application and a topical application would have little if no effect. The word lupin however, comes from the Latin lupinus meaning wolf-like. The plant has associations with the moon, imagination and unconscious. I think it is likely therefore, that it features in these types of remedies for these folkloric associations rather than any actual medicinal properties.

'Ashthroat – This is possibly vervain (*Verbena oficinalis*) and is another herb with a long and magical history and still very much in use as a nervine with a wide application for muscular spasm, nervousness, migraines, insomnia, anxiety states, exhaustion and depression. Another alternative might be Alkanet (*Anchusa officinalis*) which is not used today as far as I know but extracted into a fatty medium it releases a red colour which would stain the skin when applied and may have some ritual significance.

'Henbane (*Hyoscyamus niger*) – This plant is used primarily as an antispasmodic with particular application to the urinary system. Additionally, it is a hypnotic, sedative and a mydriadic. So it will cause relaxation and promote sleep. It has use in treating some types of headaches, neuralgia, excitability, panic, restlessness and insomnia. It is one of a number of herbs that is currently for practitioner use only and the dose has to be very carefully controlled for internal use.

'Harewort – This may refer to Mullein (*Verbascum thapsus*) or Cudweed (*Filago germanica*.) Mullein has properties and uses similar to Althaea and modern herbalists use it both internally and externally for its mucilaginous content which soothes both skin and mucous membranes particularly those of the respiratory system. It has also expectorant properties so would be of use in respiratory infections generating copious mucus. But to achieve the greatest benefits to the respiratory system presumably the plant would have to be taken internally. Cudweed is very little used but is antitussive, anti-catarrhal and antiseptic so would be used to treat upper respiratory infections and irritations if used internally.

'Whortleberry (Bilberry) (*Vaccinium myrtillus*) – The main actions here are astringency and reducing inflammation for healing wounds and ulcers. I don't know of anyone using the shoots but the fruits are being consumed for the vitamin C and A content, and commonly used as a tonic for the venous system.

'Hedgerive – This could be either Clivers (*Galium aparine*) or Burdock (*Arctium lappa*) both of which are still in use. Clivers is mostly used internally but externally it has refridgerant and demulcent actions and can be used for burns, abrasions, softening of cysts and abscesses and as an anti-hemorrhagic that could be used to stem bleeding and seal the surface. Burdock has a long use as a skin herb with antibacterial, anti-fungal and demulcent actions. So it could be used for acne, infected abrasions or wounds, boils or abscesses or infections like impetigo or styes. This might be the rationale of applying the salve to the eyes.

'Corn Cockle (*Agrostemma githago*) – This is not used today and you would have difficulty finding it, it has become so rare. In the past though it was a common weed of crops and there were reports of poisoning from the seeds contaminating flour.

'Fennel (*Foeniculum vulgare*) – This plant is aromatic, carminative and has antimicrobial actions. There are two main areas of modern use, internally as a digestive aid to reduce colic and wind, and more relevant to the remedy, as a compress for the eyes to reduce inflammation and to treat conditions like blepharitis and conjunctivitis.'

Susan has identified from her investigation of these herbs that although there are a number that would indeed act as anti-convulsive, relaxant and soporific, the plants would need to be ingested for these attributes to be successful. Lupin for example, as Susan notes, would have little if no affect when applied topically in a salve. Explaining further regarding the topical application of this remedy she says:

> 'In none of the remedies is there mention of quantities or proportions of constituents, some of which would have been active on the skin surface while others are clearly intended to be absorbed and have an effect on the nervous system. The lack of information about relative quantities of herbs and fat leaves doubt about how effective the ones intended for their internal actions would have been. However, the French herbalist Maurice Messegue successfully treated his patients with hand and footbaths only, achieving uptake though the skin. Even handling dandelion leaves is enough to stimulate diuresis, an action enshrined in the country name "wet a bed" and the French "pissenlit".'

Although some uptake of properties through the skin may thus occur, it is unlikely that this remedy was intended as an anti-convulsive for epilepsy, so it seems safe to conclude that we are indeed dealing with a category of remedy that nonetheless contains lupin, but is not intended for epilepsy. Susan also suggests that the inclusion of plants such as lupin may therefore be for their folkloric properties alone.

A more protective, amuletic character then continues into the ritualistic directives that include putting the herbs under an alter, the saying of Mass over them, the use of holy salt and just for good measure, throwing the plants into running water. If this was not enough then smoking (smudging) is also recommended. Smoking refers to herbs such as sage being used to billow smoke around a person to cleanse them of evil spirits and negative energy. Finally, 'the sign' is to be made over the person, often. This sign is probably the cross. Smearing the salve upon the eyes and face may also be protective in nature.

It has been argued by L. Kayton in *The Relationship of the Vampire to Schizophrenia* (1972) that:

> 'The specifics of the vampire legend bear a close resemblance to fundamental dynamic issues seen in schizophrenia and in the content of certain nightmares.'

Kayton identifies a number of similarities between the observed behaviours of some schizophrenics such as starvation, gorging, reversal of the day-night cycle and preoccupations with death as evidence that the vampire myth, the nightwalker perhaps, may be related to schizophrenia.

The phantasy of nocturnal, often sexual, visitations as indicated by succubae have also been linked in studies to the type of psychopathology encountered by the schizophrenic. The psychologist Richard Noll describes cases where delusional schizophrenics link sexual gratification and lust with the consumption of blood. He coined the term Renfield's Syndrome from the character Renfield in Bram Stoker's *Dracula*, and uses it to describe those who believe blood to have life-giving properties of immortality that manifest with the early libido at puberty.

Jensen and Poulsen have also linked schizophrenia to a further category of vampirism stating in their 2002 paper *Auto-vampirism in schizophrenia* that a 'relationship between vampirism, auto-vampirism and mental disorders has been established, especially with regard to schizophrenia'. Auto-vampirism refers to the act of eating oneself and although these categories of vampirism are contemporary, it could be that these characteristics existed as the nightwalkers in Old English remedies.

The notion of nightwalkers and vampires may seem fanciful today yet it might be uncomfortable to learn that the efficacy of using human blood to increase longevity is not pure fiction. Preliminary research published in the *New Scientist* in August 2014 causes one to pause and wonder whether the vampiric folklore embodied in the character Renfield's statement that 'the blood is the life', has not been stating something uncomfortably real:

> 'Giving young human blood plasma to older people with a medical condition – is about to begin. Getting approval to perform the experiment in humans has been relatively simple, thanks to the long safety record of blood transfusions. So in early October, a [team] will give a transfusion of blood plasma donated by people under 30 to older volunteers with mild to moderate Alzheimer's. Following the impressive results in animal experiments, the team hopes to see immediate improvements in cognition, [but] cautions that it is still very experimental. "We will assess cognitive function immediately before and for several days after the transfusion, as well as tracking each person for a few months to see if any of their family or carers report any positive effects. The effects might be transient, but even if it's just for a day it is a proof of concept that is worth pursuing."'

The first successful blood transfusion occurred in 1665, with the first human transfusion in 1667. Transfusing blood was a step up from consuming blood. Digestion and its resultant process of absorption has been known for centuries, yet the circulation of blood was only discovered in 1628 by the British physician William Harvey. The ancient instinct that blood was central to health, however, was certainly correct.

Since the time of the Greek physician Hippocrates (c. 450 BC), illness in the classical world was thought to be caused by an imbalance of the humours – black bile, yellow bile, phlegm and blood; the drinking and letting of blood was therefore encouraged as a general healing process for many ailments and as a rejuvenation tonic. Romans drank the blood of fallen gladiators, believing that the strength and life force of the gladiator would serve as a healthful tonic. Drinking blood was a recommended prescription in the Middle Ages. Perhaps the most famous case of blood drinking allegedly occurred in 1492, when Pope Innocent VIII drank the blood of three young boys.

The remedies against nightwalkers may imply schizophrenia, although it is uncomfortably unclear whether the intention behind such cures would have been to protect a patient from schizophrenic episodes or rather, to protect others from a perceived threat from the schizophrenic themselves.

Before leaving schizophrenia behind it is interesting to note, however, that some researchers such as Joseph Campbell have contended that our ancestors may have had a rather more positive view of what we today term schizophrenia. If correct, then his argument makes it less likely that these particularly dark nocturnal remedies point exclusively to schizophrenia.

Campbell argues in his book, *Myths to Live By* (1973), that today's schizophrenic receives little if any help in negotiating the realms of the unconscious. Contemporary psychology approaches the schizophrenic from the position of current ideas of what constitutes normality, viewing sufferers through a lens of societal norms that do not tolerate such differences. Our ancestors, on the other hand, may have viewed symptoms such as hearing voices as a divine gift that would have marked them out as having special abilities suited to work as a shaman and healer.

Campbell contends that a particular type of schizophrenia, which he terms 'essential schizophrenia', is in fact a powerful opportunity for an individual to delve into their unconscious and re-emerge, given the right support, transformed. Drawing upon the work of the late Dr John Perry, he suggests that the psychosis be allowed to run its course as a journey of self exploration through imagination. The aim being to discover aspects of one's psyche that have become lost or fragmented and by doing so, enable deep psychological healing. South African researcher Niyati Evers supports this view in her paper *Shamanic Perspectives on Mental Illness, for Pre-Modern Peoples* (2015), stating that:

> 'the schizophrenic's reason and senses, like those of the shaman during initiation, are assaulted by concrete revelations of the heights and depths of the vast Otherworlds of the collective unconscious.'

The schizophrenic is thus being likened by Campbell and Evers to the shamans of old, who recognised that seeing non-physical material and hearing voices was symptomatic of the gifts required for healing. If these 'gifts' are viewed as aberrant, then the schizophrenic becomes an unwitting victim of these otherworldly experiences which may manifest as delusions and anxieties.

Campbell is careful to differentiate essential schizophrenia from its paranoid form. Paranoid schizophrenia, he suggests, has a very specific difference in that unconscious content is projected out into the world becoming a source of threat for the sufferer. With no opportunity for internal process, this form of the illness creates such crisis that control of the symptoms is often the only medical recourse. It is possible that the leechbook remedies citing general madness, lunacy, frenzy and mania could be intended to control the phenomenology of hallucinations, delusions, dreams and chaotic speech within paranoid schizophrenia that can also resemble the manic episodes of bipolar disorder. But there is a further possibility for the nightwalker. The inclusion of succubae together with the therapeutic method of smoking a patient offer evidence for an ailment so terrifying it continues to be investigated by leading psychiatrists today.

The act of smoking or smudging utilises the olfactory process and renders the conventional applications of medicines as either internal or external defunct. When soporific calming herbs are wafted about a person before bed, this could have helped facilitate a good night's sleep. Sleeping well would have been beneficial for many illnesses of course, yet, with betony and lupin's specific folkloric connection to the moon, unconsciousness and dreams along with the general protective elements of nightwalker remedies, all aspects now combine to offer a reasonable attempt at a cure for night terrors.

Although night terrors are discussed in detail in the following chapter, suffice it to say here that The London Clinic identifies night terrors as non-normal dreams. This may not sound particularly scary, yet sufferers complain of quite terrifying experiences that feel utterly real. In a paralysed state between waking and sleeping, they report many instances of believing they are being crushed, feeling as if 'something' evil is in the room and far more. Today we know what is happening and can even identify at what point in the sleep cycle these experiences occur. For our ancestors, however, this must have been truly terrifying, and although we know that no evil vampire/nightwalker is really stalking us in our sleep, they did not.

Chapter 10

Hags *et al*

Nocturnal trauma is a unifying characteristic of three creatures – the hag, nightwalker and succubae. All three feature in the manuscripts and I suggest present nuanced facets of a singular ancient archetype associated with primal fears regarding death and repressed sexual impulses. By mythologising these fears within a working mythology of otherworldly creatures and rituals, it may be argued that the Old English folk-healer's understanding of mental health and the unconscious mind was unsurpassed until Freud and Jung.

Archetypes, as understood within psychology refer to a mental image – in this case the hag, succubae or nightwalker – that is used to interpret commonalities of behaviours and observations within our experiences. We often talk in terms of archetypes when we describe someone as a typical rebel, for example. What we mean is that we have interpreted their characteristics as being representative of a certain category of individual which can be traced back through time by association. This can lead to the habit of labelling people, viewing archetypes therefore as fixed. Jung was quite clear, however, that archetypes are always variable and it is this quality of variability that draws together the creatures under discussion and enables consideration of their potential originating mythic pathology. Marie Louise Von Franz describes how archetypal stories and characters originate:

> 'Through individual experiences of an invasion by some unconscious content, either in a dream or in a waking hallucination – some event or some mass-hallucination whereby

> an archetypal content breaks into individual life … and becomes amplified by any other existing folklore which will fit it.'
>
> (*Interpretation of Fairytales*, 1970)

The hag, nightwalker and succubae all fit Von Franz's evolution of an archetype, breaking through from the unconscious and projecting our deepest fears onto imagined monsters. These bizarre and forgotten Old English characters then emerge from 'unconscious content' linked to hallucinatory dream state attacks that in turn became embodied and amplified in folklore from the Middle East to Northern Europe.

We encountered the Old English hag (*Hægtesse*) within the charm for a sudden stitch. The charm, which called upon further feminine characters such as mighty women (*mihtigan wif*) to protect against the shot from hags, contains one of the few specific references to hags that we find in ancient texts.

The root of the word hag can be traced as far back as the proto-Germanic language which evolved into the Elder Futhark, the oldest of runic alphabets. The proto-Germanic word is *hagatusjon* that evolved into many forms such the Old High German word *hagzissa,* which means hex. *Haghetisse* in Dutch and *haugtusse* in Norwegian both mean a woman who dwells beneath the earth, something akin to a goblin.

The identity of the hag within folklore has become distorted and generalised over time. In the charm for a sudden stitch, the term *hægtessan gescot* (hag's shot) is commonly translated as witch's shot, evidencing how the terms witch and hag have become synonymous with each other today. Witches are generally viewed as having hag-like features of hook noses, warts and green skin. At Halloween, we see the old hag remembered in the modern witch as hoards of children march the streets knocking upon doors demanding 'trick or treat', a custom so evocative of their impoverished English ancestors who would beg door to door for spiced soul cakes on All Souls' Day offering prayers for the dead.

Before All Souls' Day existed, however, the druidic festival of Samhain marked the days from October 31 to November 2. For three nights, people would put candles at every opening within their home and children would beg at each door for alms. Samhain was a time when the Druids believed the world of the dead moved closer to our own and this belief, although comforting for those whose loved ones had passed, evoked fear also. The dead could not always be trusted. Dark creatures could also use this opaque time to draw near and steal the souls of the living. Superstition fuelled the belief, therefore, that Samhain was a time for hags, nightwalkers and all things evil.

Despite being synonymous with the word witch today, it is possible, however, to tease out characteristics of the hag that have arisen in response to a specific human experience. In folkloric belief, the hag sits upon the chest of a person, sucking their life force whilst they sleep. The victim may experience this as a particularly bad nightmare leaving them tired the next day. The modern phrase 'hag-ridden' is sometimes used to describe the feeling of sleep deprivation.

Hag visitations are not always contained to the phenomenon of nightmares and fatigue, however, as some have reported actual sightings of the hag herself, sitting on their chest, drinking in their energy whilst they themselves are paralysed and suffocated by her weight. In Persia, this nocturnal visitor was called Bakhtak and in Scandinavia her name was Mare. Lilith from the Old Testament was also such a creature. Sometimes the hag was thought to be the soul of a sinfully damned woman returning in death to traumatise the living, and in this guise, she was known as a succubae which would have no choice but to survive upon the stolen life force of others. The hag and succubae may therefore be two faces of the same creature.

The hag as a bringer of nightmares together with feelings of weight, paralysis, suffocation and hallucinations fulfils the medical requirements for the condition known as sleep paralysis. Sleep paralysis, which includes within its pathology the phenomenon of night terrors, is particularly unsettling as it often involves waking into consciousness before the brain has informed the body, resulting in an unpleasant situation where one is awake yet unable to move. Patients also describe feeling a weight upon their chest or of being smothered, combined with the feeling that something malevolent is in the room.

Hallucinations can add to the experience, with victims actually seeing terrifying old women. To the waking mind, these creatures are experienced as real.

Symptoms associated with sleep paralysis result from the transition stages between sleep and waking becoming disjointed. The term Old Hag Syndrome continues to be used to describe the condition.

Old Hag Syndrome is understood today in neuroscience. It is thought to be a glitch in the firing of neurons that can occur to varying degrees when a subject transitions from sleep to wakefulness. The brain fails to let the body know it is awake and so the dream state continues into the conscious realm. The subject then experiences these hallucinations from the unconscious mind as every bit as real as normal daytime phenomena.

Consultant psychiatrist and sleep specialist, Dr Nik Gkampranis, told me that sleep paralyisis is 'the inability to speak, move or react occurring when a person falls off to sleep or awakens. Though it is temporary and passes within seconds or minutes it can be extremely frightening for the person experiencing it.' He goes on to explain that of itself, the condition is not harmful, although further symptoms such as sensations of choking, hallucinations and an 'impending sense of doom' can present as part of other disorders such as narcolepsy, anxiety, depression and insomnia. Regarding cause, Dr Gkampranis says:

> 'The exact pathophysiology of sleep is unknown but it is thought that sleep paralysis occurs when a person experiences rapid eye movement (REM) sleep whilst being awake. During REM sleep the muscles are paralysed with exemption the muscles of the eyes and respiration muscles. When the patient awakes from REM sleep it is likely that the muscles are not active yet and those few seconds can present as sleep paralysis.'

Dr Gkampranis diagnoses the condition via a sleep study (polysomnography) and although specific treatment is unnecessary, 'Good sleep hygiene and improving sleep habits are the mainstay' along with treating any underlying sleep disorders or psychiatric conditions.

For our ancestors, these extreme experiences must have been utterly terrifying and, unlike a physical disease that could be explained by the arrows of elves, hags were considered the culprits for nightmarish encounters. An apparent mystery remains, however, as neuroscience struggles to explain why sufferers who have no previous knowledge of sleep paralysis or the Old Hag Syndrome continue to see hags in their hallucinations. Furthermore, accounts have been forwarded that suggest the hags have at times been witnessed by third parties. Occultist Montague Summers and Dr Franz Hartmann, both interested in supernatural phenomena reported the unusual nineteenth century case of a servant boy who was recently employed by a miller:

> '[The] miller had a healthy servant-boy, who soon after entering his service began to fail. He acquired a ravenous appetite, but nevertheless grew daily more feeble and emaciated. Being interrogated, he at last confessed that a thing which he could not see, but which he could plainly feel, came to him every night about twelve o'clock and settled upon his chest, drawing all the life out of him, so that he became paralysed for the time being, and neither could move nor cry out. Thereupon the miller agreed to share the bed with the boy, and made him promise that he should give a certain sign when the vampire arrived. This was done, and when the signal was made the miller putting out his hands grasped an invisible but very tangible substance that rested upon the boy's chest. He described it as apparently elliptical in shape, and to the touch feeling like gelatin, properties which suggest an ectoplasmic formation. The thing writhed and fiercely struggled to escape, but he gripped it firmly and threw it on the fire. After that the boy recovered, and there was an end of these visits.'

There is no research to validate this type of data and the flaws in testimony are clear, but this personal experience is still ethnographically interesting and identified by Summers as being typical of the material reported by victims of so called vampire and hag attacks. This typical material begins to create an archetype where nocturnal experiences of being paralysed, perhaps one could also say enchanted whilst a creature sucks life force or blood, pull together motifs common to both hags and vampires indicating that there might well be a prior archetypal creature from which both emerged.

The personal subjective data in Summers' report points to the interior psychological experience showing how these supernatural characters are really unconscious content. Jung believed that a supernatural encounter with such identities was evidence of an archetypal experience and when a number of individuals experience synchronicitous phenomena, this is because the archetype exists in what he came to term the 'collective unconscious' of humanity.

Current research reveals just how real these types of night terror phenomena can seem. An unusual occurrence was relayed by Wayne King in the *New York Times* of 10 May 1981. He reported on the mysterious deaths of eighteen people who were in good health, yet all died at the same time in the early hours whilst asleep. Although their deaths remain a mystery, it has been speculated by medical practitioners that nightmares might have been the cause. This means that they were frightened to death in their sleep, or during the transitioning period. This has led to a new category of sleep disorder called Nightmare Death Syndrome, where the victim dies during sleep or the transitory stages of sleep due to nothing other than fright.

Death is a subject plagued by mystery and it is unsurprising that many myths and supernatural beliefs have emerged in an attempt to assuage the fears inherent in this mostly unknown and seemingly inevitable process. Hags may be an embodiment of these transitional fears where the ultimate fear of death emerges from the unconscious as a hag or vampire encounter. Nightwalkers (*nihtgengan)* and shadowwalkers (*sceadugengan*) may be related creatures or an emergent development from the notion of the hag. Either way, their characteristics are remarkably similar to the hag and vampire, further hinting at a potential common archetype that most probably arose from humanity's enduring fear of death and complex experiences of somnambulant phenomena. As Von Franz states:

> 'The vampire motif is world-wide … Their lust for blood is the craving or impulse of the unconscious contents to break into consciousness. If they are denied they begin to drain energy from consciousness, leaving the individual fatigued and listless.'

We have seen two remedies against nightwalkers previously, both of which displayed defensiveness and suggested a potential explanation of night terrors. Although hags were not mentioned in the remedy, the inclusion of people having sex with the devil (succubae) could be argued as having inferred their presence.

Succubae are common to myths stretching back thousands of years and their sexual behaviour is similar to that of the British Hag, the Irish Banshee and the Nightwalker. She seduces her victim, often while they sleep, draining their life force and blood and forcing them to copulate with her. The Old Irish *Dearg-Dul*, a possible relation of the Banshee, would appear as a beautiful woman to lure and seduce its victim with the sexual act before drinking their blood. Disguised as a beautiful woman this may not seem so bad but once the act is complete her true hag-like identity is revealed.

Stephen Pollington suggests a *Lacnunga* remedy against 'elf-siden and all temptations of the (fiend) devil' (*ælfidene ond wiđ eallum feondes costungum*), is also referring to the earlier belief in succubae:

> 'This complaint may be, as some have thought, the terrifying 'nightmare' but is possibly a nocturnal, sexual fantasy similar to the incubus and succubus of classical pagan thought.'

It could be suggested that the characters of the hag, vampire/nightwalker and succubae are all facets of a similar archetype that acts as a repository for some of our deepest impulses, fears and experiences. Rodriguez de la Sierra explains in his 1998 paper *Origin of the myth of vampirism*:

> 'The significance and universal persistence of the myth suggests deep roots in the evolution of our psyche. It suggests the omnipresent desire to conquer the secret of life while containing the elements of its renewal. It represents the terrible desire for survival, destroying others to maintain his own existence … Vampirism, as a mortal sin, is contained in the image that most often comes to mind, the perverse *nature* of the vampiric act, in which the bite and the sucking of blood produce an orgasmic sensation which supersedes coitus.'

There is one primal mythic and literary character that may fit the descriptions of hag, nightwalker and succubae. In doing so, it perhaps offers a route to the genesis of this archetype before it became dispersed into the wider categories of our three protagonists used within the Old English remedies to describe unconscious mental content and subsequent nocturnal trauma. This potential prior singular archetype is Lilith.

Lilith is an ancient Sumerian and Babylonian goddess or perhaps more accurately, demoness. In old Hebrew, her name translates as 'night-hag' and she appears in many texts including the Bible, the Dead Sea Scrolls (Songs of the Sage) and the Babylonian Talmud. Curiously, however, she surfaces in one of the most famous Old English poems – *Beowulf* – as the ancestor of the monster Grendel and his mother.

Beowulf is written in Old English around the same time or slightly earlier than Bald's *Leechbook*. The story itself is likely transcribed from an older oral version which, although set in Scandinavia, was written down in England, probably by first or second generation settlers during the Dark Ages. In brief, the part of the poem we are concerned with tells the story of the hero Beowulf, a Swede who comes to the aid of the Danish King Hrothgar, whose people have been attacked at night in their mead hall by a terrible monster called Grendel. The king's men had been powerless against the fiend but when Beowulf arrived, he lay awake awaiting the creature and sure enough, when all was still, Grendel appeared and Beowulf pounced;

so great was the hero's strength that he ripped Grendel's arm clean off and the monster retreated in fear. There was much celebration, but what was unknown was the fury of a mother – Grendel's mother who captured and killed one of the king's advisors in revenge. The people were terrified of this new threat, so Beowulf agreed to fight and kill Grendel's mother in the swamp where she lived and following a terrible battle, Beowulf seized a magic sword from her own cave and slew her.

In line 1259 we read Grendel's mother (*Grendles mōdor*) described as an *ides aglæc-wif. Wif* means wife or woman, although Frederick Klaeber in his 1922 book *Beowulf and the Fight at Finnsburg* translated it as monster, wretch or demon. The common identity of Grendel's mother as a monstrous demonic female is generally considered correct and most translators follow this tradition. However, *ides* means a dignified and respected woman in Old English, Old High German and Old Saxon, and has been linked to the term Valkyrie by Rudolf Simek and directly compared to the *mihtigan wif* (mighty women) in the charm for a sudden stitch by researcher Dr Hilda Davidson. Helen Damico argues in her essay, *The Valkyrie Reflex in Old English Literature*, (1980) that:

> 'In both their benevolent and malevolent aspects, the valkyries are related to a generic group of half-mortal, half-supernatural beings called idisi in Old High German, ides in Old English, and dis in Old Norse, plural, disir. Both groups are closely allied in aspect and function: they are armed, powerful, priestly. The Beowulf poet follows the tradition of depicting the valkyrie-figure as a deadly battle demon in his characterization of Grendel's Mother. As Chadwick has argued, Grendel's Mother, that wælgæst wæfre 'roaming slaughter-spirit' epitomizes the earlier concept of the valkyrie.'

Klaeber acknowledges that the translation of *aglæc* as monster is contentious and may have had a dual meaning for our ancestors. He notes that certain occurrences of the word within the text (such as line

893) may actually refer to Beowulf rather than Grendel, leading Klaeber to concur with Doreen Gillam (1961) that *aglæc* may mean fierce fighter as well as monster. This is not the first fluidity of identity between good/bad hero/monster that we find in the poem. At the beginning, when Grendel first goes to the mead-hall, both Grendel and Beowulf are described as *hefiche* which means mighty one. In fact, it is not easy at times to differentiate whether the narrator is describing Grendel or Beowulf. So, is Grendel's mother a monstrous night-hag or a dignified warrior woman, or can she be both? To answer this question, we must go back further in time to trace the genealogy of Grendel's mother.

We learn within Beowulf that Grendel and his mother are of the bloodline of Cain:

> *'Wæs se grimma gæst Grendel hāten, Mære mearc-stapa, sē þe mōras hēold, Fen ond fæsten; fīfel-cynnes eard Won-sæli wer weardode hwīle, Siþðan him Scyppend forscrifen hæfde In Caines cynne þone cwealm gewræc Ēce Drihten, þæs þe hē Ābel slōg. Ne gefeah hē þære fæhðe, ac hē hine feor forwræc, Metod for þy māne, man-cynne fram. Þanon untydras ealle onwōcon, Eotenas ond ylfe ond orcnēas, Swylce gīgantas, þā wið Gode wunnon.*
>
> 'This ghastly demon was called Grendel walker of the marshes he who held the moors, fen and desolate stronghold; the land of marsh creatures, the wretched creature ruled for a time since him the creator had condemned with Cain's kin, that killing avenged the eternal Lord, in which he slew Abel; this feud he did not enjoy, and drove him far away, the Ruler for his crime, from mankind; then awful offspring all awoke, ogres and elves underworld spirits, also giants, who with god battled.'

As well as providing further fascinating insight into the mythology of our ancestors and the basis for their psychological remedies we learn that by virtue of Cain's bloodline, Grendel's mother is a descendent of the night-hag Lilith. In the Old Testament, we learn that Lilith was thrown out of Eden because she was disobedient and would not be subservient to her husband Adam. She was thus cast out in preference of Eve and changed by God into a demon. With her new husband, Cain, she gave birth to a legion of demons and monsters with the *Beowulf* poet stating that all fearsome creatures of the underworld, elves and ogres, evil spirits and giants are descendants of these first lovers.

One of the earliest references to Lilith can be found written upon two seventh century BC Babylonian incantation bowls that were used for exorcising, conjuring and in some cases trapping demons. One of the bowls, which was discovered in the ancient Sumerian city of Nippur, depicts Lilith with her long wild hair, reminiscent of the flaming wild hair of her children, the *Lamiae* (another English name for vampire). Surrounding her is Aramaic text that forms a magical incantation of a binding charm and exorcism. Such a charm would have been used to prevent Lilith from doing harm and translates as follows:

> 'You are bound and sealed, all you demons and devils and liliths, by that hard and strong, mighty and powerful bond with which are tied Sison… The evil Lilith, who causes the hearts of men to go astray and appears in the dream of the night and in the vision of late day.
>
> 'Who burns and casts down with nightmare, attacks and kills children, boys and girls.
>
> 'She is conquered and sealed away from the house and from the threshold of Bahram-Gushnasp son of Ishtar-Nahid by the talisman of Metatron, the great prince who is called the Great Healer of Mercy.... who vanquishes demons and devils, black arts and mighty charms and keeps them away from the house and threshold.'

The spell and its interpretation are clearly intended to protect the 'house and threshold' from attack and offers us a vivid window upon the actions and traits associated with Lilith over two thousand years ago. First, we see that although Lilith was certainly known as a demon in her own right, being described within the spell in the singular, she is also presented in the plural or perhaps we could say collective as liliths, indicating a lineage or species of demon with common traits. Seduction is a further characteristic of Lilith as she leads 'the hearts of men to go astray'.

The Lilith incantation charm mentions more than once that its aim is to keep Lilith 'away from the house'. This seems to indicate that the bowl served as a protective amulet to be kept within the home to ward off hag attacks and protect the family.

An interesting piece of information usually disregarded by researchers, however, is that these particular bowls were not found within the remains of a settlement as we would expect; they were found, instead, buried with the dead in an ancient pre-Christian cemetery. It is probable, given the text, that the charm did at one time serve to protect a household or individual within the home, but when a death occurred, it seems protection was required for the recently deceased also.

In the Occidental world, Lilith morphed in belief with Hecate who is often described as awaiting weary travelers at crossroads before attacking them and feeding on their blood. Often considered a Hellenic goddess, Hecate's roots stretch further back into the ancient past and she may even be a proto-Lilith. She is mentioned in Turkey in the sixth century BC and was worshipped earlier than this in the North and Asia Minor during the eighth century BC and her identity has changed as she has journeyed through the belief structures of different cultures. By the time she reached Aegina, an island off Greece and the centre of her cult during Hellenistic times, she had become one face of a triune goddess called upon by humanity to intercede where all else had failed. Hecate was the face of the night, Circe was a beautiful temptress and their sister Medea was known for weaving and divination.

There is evidence, however, that Hecate's character was not always so darkly defined as, early in her worship, she was sought as the nourisher of babies and her counsel was thought to be wise and just.

In prehistoric times, she was thus viewed in less black and white terms and seen more as a force of nature capable of both dark and light, creativity and destruction. The same may be true of Lilith who was once the good child of God.

A document discovered in the Nag Hammadhi library dated to 350 BC called *Thunder Perfect Mind* points to this pre-biblical goddess. It is an extraordinary paradoxical monologue, spoken by a female deity who states that she is the first and the last, the whore and the holy one, the mother and the daughter. Her teaching continues in this dualistic style, forcing a perspective where light collapses into the landscape of darkness and good cannot exist without evil. Hecate once existed as the embodiment of both. She was liminal and associated with crossings and boundaries, as was Grendel.

Grendel himself is described as a boundary-stepper. *Sceadu* means shadow in Old English and *genga* means walker or goer. In the line 703 we read – *Com on wanre niht, scrīðan sceadu-genga* (came on a dark night, gliding, a shadow-walker). *Scrīðan* meaning 'to glide' is also very similar to the word *Scrīfan* which means that a person's fate is determined. So, this gliding is not just a method of supernatural transportation, Grendel isn't just light on his feet. The wording conjures a creature moving towards its prey in a manner that is fated and therefore, beyond the human being's conscious control. Grendel and his kind are certainly creatures of the night described in further passages as *mære* which means night-monster and in Modern English, nightmare. Lilith is also described as a creature of nightmares on the incantation bowls.

Let us consider the following passage from the poem:

'Wæs se grimma gæst Grendel haten, mære mearcstapa, se þe moras heold, fen ond fæsten; fifelcynnes eard.

'Grendel this monster grim was called, boundary-stepper mighty, in moorland dwelled, in fen and fastness; land of the giants.'

In the second line, we see the word, boundary-stepper. This is my translation of the Old English word *mearcstapa*. It is most usually translated as march-stepper. However, whilst the word *stapa* does indeed mean to step, the word *mearc* means mark or boundary and usually referred to boundary markers and signs, the points or symbols that mark one space from another, or the crossing of paths. Grendel and his kind are therefore liminal creatures spanning the boundaries of conscious and unconscious experiences, forcing repressed content to erupt into monstrous nocturnal somnambulant attacks.

British vampire folklore has always been believed to be an import from Europe and the Far East, with vampires only reaching Britain with the literature of the nineteenth century. It could be suggested that this view requires revision as the nightwalkers from *Lacnunga* and *Beowulf*, although not termed 'vampire', are indicative of an archetype associated with nightmares, sex, blood, sleep paralysis and death. This literary and folkloric evidence can now be combined with new archaeological burial data from England to confirm that 'vampires' known within the Old English texts therefore as nightwalkers, have indeed been here for some time.

Archaeologist Charles Daniels discovered a body dating from 550-700AD buried in Southwell, England. Its heart was ritualistically pierced by a stake, as were its hands and feet and it is now known as the Southwell Vampire. Since then, a number of further Anglo-Saxon 'vampires' have been found with stakes through their hearts. Many of these burials were ignored by archaeologists as simply being evidence of fear surrounding deviant members of society. Yet John Blair, professor of medieval history at Oxford University, has linked another twelfth century Old English document called the *Life and Miracles of Saint Modwenna* to an Anglo-Saxon belief in the walking dead. He states that such burials were a 'deliberate decisive measure, to keep this person down in the grave so they can never walk around again.'

Also writing in the twelfth century, Geoffrey of Burton documents a curious case in the small English village of Drakelow, where villagers reported seeing two recently deceased men carrying their own coffins through the village lanes and fields bringing disease to all who encountered them. Three people died and 'men were living in terror of the phantom dead men'. It was decided therefore, following permission from the bishop, that the men's bodies should be dug up so their hearts could be removed and their heads cut off. The hearts and heads were then carried across running water and the phantoms ceased. (quoted in Bartlett, 2002).

The Old English hag may therefore stand alongside the succubae and nightwalkers from Bald's *Leechbook III* and *Lacnunga* as embodiments of an ancient archetype identifying extreme nocturnal experiences we term sleep paralysis and night terrors. As an archetype, her psychological heritage forms a mythic landscape used by our ancestors to understand these terrifying nighttime phenomena and cultivate remedies, rituals and narratives to effect healing or at the very least, a reduction in symptoms.

The liminal quality of these creatures that span between the conscious and unconscious can be seen expressed within conflicting identities. The hag can sometimes appear as a young, beautiful woman and the potential genesis of this archetype, Hecate, was once viewed as a nurturing life giving goddess. Light can, therefore, become dark in the fate of old beliefs as new deities evolve and corrupt the old. Similarly, and with a strange synchronicity, the Old English healers from whom these remedies were collected became victims of a similar fate.

Chapter 11

'Cunning-Women'

The remaining mystery of Bald's *Leechbook III* and *Lacnunga* must be the identities of the healers themselves. Who were these people mixing herbs, battling nightwalkers and prescribing that women jump dead men's graves? That they existed is obvious and faint voices may be heard emerging from the texts. Yet these voices can be amplified by drawing on evidence from further disciplines such as archaeology and literature to present a portrait of a unique class of female healers whose presence has been wiped from the historic record.

To unravel the lost story of who these women healers were and begin to ask the difficult question regarding why their presence became lost to the world, a particulalrly female remedy serves to introduce their living reality. If one imagines journeying a few hundred years into the past, women can be heard here, talking about the things women often need to talk about:

> *'Wiþ þon þe wif ne mæge bearn acennan nim feldmoran nioþowearde, wyl on meolcum ond on wætre, do begea emfela, sele etan þa moran ond þæt wos supan. To þon olcan bind on þæt winstre þeoh up wið þæt cennende lim nioþowearde beolonan oþþe xii corn cellendran sædes ond þæt sceal don cniht oððe mæden. Swa þæt bearn sie acenned do þa wyrta aweg py læs þæt innelfe utsige. Gif of wife nelle gan æfter þam beorþre þæt gecyndelic sie, seope eald spic on wætre, beþe mid þone cwip oððe hleomoc oþþe hocces leaf wyl on ealoþ, sele drincan hit hat. Gif on wife sie dead bearn wyl on meolce ond on wætre hleomoc ond polleian, sele drincan on dæg tuwa.*

Georne is to wyrnanne bearneacnum wife þæt hio aht sealtes ete oððe swetes, oppe beor drince, ne swines flæac ete, ne naht fætes, ne of hire sie ær riht tide. Gif hio blede to swiþe æfter þam beorþre nioþowearde clatan wyl on meolce, sele etan ond supan þæt wos.'

'If a woman is unable to bear a child, take wild parsnip root, boil it in milk and in water, add equal amounts of both, give the roots to eat and the juice to sip. For the same, bind on the left thigh, up against the genital area, the lower part of henbane or twelve grains of coriander seed, and a boy or girl must do it; as the child is born, take the plants away lest the innards come out. If what is natural will not go out of a mother after the birth, boil old lard in water, bathe with it the vulva, or with speedwell or leaf of hock, boil it in ale, give it to drink hot. If a dead child be in her, boil in milk and in water speedwell, and pennyroyal, give it to drink twice a day. Earnestly one must refuse a pregnant woman that she should eat anything salty, nor anything sweet, nor drink beer, nor eat pig's flesh, nor anything fatty, nor drink till she be drunk, nor travel afar, nor ride too vigorously on a horse, lest the baby come away from her before the right time. If she should bleed too much after the childbirth, boil burdock root in milk, give it to eat and the broth to drink.'

A ninth century healer, when asked what she would recommend for the process of childbirth, might recount a list such as we find above. Each stage of pregnancy is covered here. The first part of the list concerns infertility, or difficulty conceiving and maintaining a pregnancy. Parsnip is recommended here as the main medicinal ingredient. Known for its health benefits, particularly during pregnancy due to its high levels of folic acid and B vitamins, parsnip is an appropriate and safe remedy. Folic acid has been shown to decrease the likelihood of birth defects as well as aiding the healthy growth of children. Symbolically, parsnip also resembles the phallus.

The next part of the list is less clear. Henbane taken internally has been used in the past for pain relief and forms the basis of certain medicines today. Modern applications are carefully regulated and are not recommended for pregnant women as henbane is toxic. The herb contains hyoscyamine and scopolamine that aid muscle relaxation, which is why henbane was also used in the past for menstrual cramping. There is no reason why binding it to the thigh would serve any physical purpose, so we must look to folkloric or magical interpretation for a possible answer.

There is an ancient creation belief that was commonly known to our ancestors, and illustrations concerning it appear in a number of old herbals and texts. The story, emerging from ancient Egypt tells that the first created human was a hermaphrodite, with a penis on the right thigh and a vagina on the left. When the thighs were rubbed together, this being created further beings, separate from the creator god. It may be that attaching henbane to the left thigh, the area where the symbolic vagina occurs, was thought to sympathetically promote pain relief.

The second part of the remedy concerns the placenta and what to do if it does not detach naturally following the birth. Here we are told to make a warm drink and bathe the vulva, both of which would have had a soothing effect. Also, hock is part of the mallow family and the Anglo-Saxons used mallow to draw out impurities from the skin such as splinters and infections when used as a poultice. A poultice of mallow may have been thought to aid, sympathetically, the drawing out of the placenta and the drink may have acted to this effect internally. Mallow is also a stomach tonic. Speedwell and its close relation, brooklime, are emmenagogues and expectorants that promote menstrual flow and therefore, this remedy may have useful for passing the placenta.

The third part of the cure concerns the removal of a foetus that has died in the womb. We see speedwell used again here but this time combined with the more powerful emmenagogue, pennyroyal. Speedwell is also an expectorant and pennyroyal has long tradition of use for abortions, so a combination of these herbs to induce early labour is logical. Pennyroyal is still used today, although it is far from safe. The quantities required to induce labour are large, large enough to also cause kidney failure, liver damage and even death. Unfortunately, women have turned to pennyroyal in the past and still do so in the present, where legal abortions are costly or unavailable. The drink would have been pleasant and minty to the taste, but pennyroyal is extremely dangerous and should not be taken.

We then come to a general list of recommendations for pregnant women. Included are useful pieces of information such as not getting drunk and to refrain from vigorous horse riding. Finally, there are directives for staunching post birth bleeding. Burdock root, also known as beggar's buttons should be boiled in milk and given as a drink. Although Burdock is known to be useful for purifying the blood, it is unlikely it would have been useful in reducing excessive post-birth bleeding.

So, who was this person recounting so useful a list as this and can we ascertain a gender? Archaeological research suggests that we can. Archaeologists specialising in Anglo-Saxon inhumations and cremations believe they have observed a pattern concerning the graves of certain females. From assessing the items within each grave such as garments, tools and further objects, researcher Audrey Meaney has theorised that these women were healers.

In her 1981 book, *Anglo-Saxon Amulets and Curing Stones*, she argues that there was a specifically female-oriented medical profession of English folk-healers who used magic and herbs to bring help and healing to local communities. She called these healers 'cunning-women' from the Old English word *cunning* meaning 'knowledgeable'. If Meaney is correct and these Anglo-Saxon burials do contain the corpses of healers, then Bald's remedies may represent their legacy and the new medical arena of Ancientbiotics where the remedy for an eye salve cures the superbug MRSA, may owe its success to English cunning-women.

Tania Dickinson explored the burial of one such female in some detail. In her paper *An Anglo-Saxon "Cunning Woman" from Bidford-on-Avon*, Dickinson specifically identifies an early Saxon burial as that of a 'cunning woman' or Old English folk-healer. The woman was discovered in 1971, oriented south-west to north-east at the edge of

Bidford-on-Avon's Anglo-Saxon cemetery and Dickinson catagorised the grave objects as fastenings for clothes, jewellery and 'objects and/or bag, suspended by the left hip'. It is this bag and related items including 'an unusual scalpel-like knife' that sparked the interest of academics leading Meaney and Dickinson to suggest that such burials are evidence of a special class of medical women. Burials of this type are predominantly found dating from the fifth to seventh centuries, although similar ones from Northern England have been found from the Middle Ages. Citing Meaney, Andrew Reynolds (*Anglo-Saxon Deviant Burial Customs* 2014) comments of these burials:

> 'Their characteristics were defined largely on the basis of the objects that they contained. Many of these special women's graves ... contain overtly amuletic objects, while others are equipped with a complex or unusual range of kit including, as indicated by iron or ivory bag rings, often containing small objects, very often of an apparently non-functional or non-utilitarian character.'

The cunning-woman of Bidford-on-Avon showed signs of wearing a long robe indicative of status and wealth within a larger graveyard of noticeably poorer people. This is not unusual, as it seems that these woman were held in high regard. Yet if one consults the accepted history of medicine, they are nowhere to be seen. This begs the question – what happened to them? The answer to this question is complex, deserving of a whole book of its own. Yet three themes arise from literary and documentary evidence that begins to solve the problem and bring light to a previously forgotten, buried past. These themes involve status, gender and religion.

Neil Carver states the point quite succinctly in his BBC article *The Anglo-Saxon Cunning Woman* (November 2012). The background to his quotation below is that Meaney's cunning-women are comparable to similar graves found in Scandinavia thus demonstrating that the role of females in healthcare was not confined to Britain:

> 'Archaeologist Neil Price has found female shamans to be important players among the Vikings – in fact, they were recorded as active all round the Arctic circle into recent times. Shamans' powers included divining the future, healing, shoring up the timorous and protecting the vulnerable – a mixture of doctor, psychiatrist, marriage councillor, midwife, politician and priest. Their prescriptions included remedial potions, laying on hands and reporting visions induced by singing and dancing – altogether not so distant from their modern successors, the doctors and the bishops of the 21st century.'

The cunning-women are identified here as shamans, a term which describes their interdisciplinary roles of physician and priest. The word 'shaman' comes from the Siberian Tungusian tribes and although today it is used to classify the generalised spiritual practices of indigenous cultures, it is clear from the lineage of persistent Siberian practice that the word designated a particular individual within the community who used herbs, song, dance, trance and supernatural abilities to help others. Carver mentions that the female shamans were recorded and the records he refers to are the great Sagas that survive from the frozen North which portray, in great detail, stories of these women, bringing them alive for the modern reader.

A particularly powerful depiction of a possible cunning-woman or shaman fitting Carver's description is retained in the Icelandic Saga of Erik the Red. The author of the tale is unknown but it is dated to just the time when Bald's book would have been commissioned and, similarly, is thought to be from an earlier work. The woman's name was Thorbiorg and although the report is situated in Greenland, anthropologists and historians believe these women would have been common throughout Europe and the British Isles.

The setting is one of despair as the northern regions were experiencing great famine and its people were feeling the onslaught of hunger and cold. One small village yeoman decided to invite a famous priestess to visit them during their winter festival, hoping she would be able to reveal the time when their suffering would cease.

Thorbiorg, said to be the last of nine great sisters (recall the nine sisters of *Noththe*), arrives at the feasting hall during the evening cloaked in deep blue. Gems line the hems of her garment, glistening along the seams right to the very ground. Her hood is of black lambskin, lined with white cats' fur and her hands are covered in cat skin gloves. Calf skin boots with brass buttons adorn her feet. She carries a great staff set with gems and around her waist is a girdle made of wood, from which hangs a large leather pouch containing herbs and other materials for working charms.

The villagers treated Thorbiorg like a priestess, and it is interesting to note that the great Roman historian Tacitus (AD 56-117), who travelled Northern Europe and the British Isles with the Roman armies recording with intricate detail all the folk customs of its peoples, wrote whilst in Germania of the reverence afforded to certain powerful women who held a place of great honour and authority in society and:

> '... according to the ancient German custom which regards many women as endowed with prophetic powers, and as the superstition grows, attributes divinity to them'.

Commanding such high social status, Thorbiorg was thus treated to a grand feast of meat, goat's cheese and the hearts of beasts despite the scarcity of food. She was invited to sit upon a throne where she was greeted and welcomed. The yeoman then asked her if she might look around the gathering of people and attest as to their worthiness. Thorbiorg responded that she was very pleased with the character of the people and that after a night's sleep, she would help the village by answering their questions regarding the future.

The following day, Thorbiorg began preparing for the ritual which would enable her to see the future. She asked the villagers to bring any local cunning-women forward to assist her with the necessary incantations and charms. Unfortunately, none could be found and so:

> 'Thereupon a search was made throughout the house, to see whether anyone knew how to recite the [incantation]. Then the

> girl Gudrid said: "Although I am neither skilled in the magic arts nor a prophetess, yet my foster-mother, Halldis, taught me in Iceland that charm-song, which she called Warlocks." Thorbiorg answered: "Then thou art wise in season!" Gudrid replied: "This is an incantation and ceremony of such a kind, that I do not intend to lend it any aid, for I am a good Christian woman. Thorbiorg answered: "It could so be that thou could give thy help to the people here, yet still be a good Christian woman; but I will leave it with Thorkel to provide for my needs."'

Thorkel, the yeoman, orders Gudrid to assist Thorbiorg with the special incantation and the ritual commences with the women of the village forming a circle with Thorbiorg at the centre, whilst Gudrid sings the incantation so beautifully that it enchants all who have gathered there. Thorbiorg is impressed by Gudrid's singing saying:

> 'She has indeed lured many spirits here who have found the song to be very pleasant to hear; those spirits who wanted to forsake us and refuse to submit themselves to us have joined us here. Many things are now revealed to me which were previously hidden, both, from me and from others. I am able to proclaim that this period of famine will not endure and the fortunes will increase as spring approaches. The visitation of disease, which has been so long upon you, will disappear sooner than expected. And thee, Gudrid, I shall reward for your assistance as your destiny has also been revealed to me. Thou shalt make a most worthy marriage here in Greenland, but it shall not be of long duration for your future path leads out to Iceland, and a lineage both great and goodly shall spring from thee, and above thy line brighter rays of light shall shine than I have power clearly to reveal. And now farewell and health to thee, my daughter!'

Following this general assurance that the difficult times would pass, Thorbiorg invited individuals from the village to approach her with their private concerns and it is told that little of what she prophesied failed to come to pass and after the ritual was finished, the great priestess continued her journey through the frozen North to attend further invitations.

Further accounts of similar women survive from elsewhere in Europe. Tacitus writes in his Germania chronicles that the Germanic tribes 'believe that there resides in women an element of holiness and a gift of prophesy' and he puts forward the example of Valeda, a Germanic priestess whom the Romans encountered during their defeat of 69AD when they had been forced by the German tribes to attempt a peaceful negotiation. Valeda held tribal authority, yet was considered far too sacred and important to appear before the Romans herself. Instead, her male attendants were used to mediate with them.

One might imagine the humiliation and insult suffered by the Roman general under such circumstances, yet women of power were not unknown to the early Mediterranean cultures either. The Greeks and Romans also viewed certain women as having a mysterious yet privileged access to a type of knowledge unknown to the wider world. Their priestesses were called *manteis*, and the *manteis* would experience visions and ecstasies in which new knowledge would emerge to enrich and illuminate embodied consciousness. However, their visionary reports were often difficult to decipher and so they would have male attendants called *prophetai* who would interpret their utterances for people to understand.

Plato termed their visionary state a 'divine frenzy', which requires an apparent loss of control akin to madness. Indeed, visionary states of ecstasy must have seemed almost identical to madness when observed. As the twelfth century writer known as Gerald of Wales describes:

> 'they immediately go into a trance and lose control of their senses, as if they are possessed. They do not answer the question put to them in a logical way. Words stream from their mouths, incoherently and apparently meaningless and without any sense at all, but all the same well expressed: and if you listen carefully

> to what they say you will receive the solution to your problem. When it is all over, they will recover from their trance, as if they were ordinary people waking from heavy sleep.'

The philosopher Socrates once stated, however, that 'our greatest blessings come to us by way of madness'. Socrates believed that true knowledge stands and speaks beyond the confines of time, requiring not just a cognitive faculty to decipher meaning within our thinking world, but also the ability to 'lose the mind' to enable such knowledge to emerge in the first place.

It is possible, therefore, that the power and prestige of these women who served as mediators with the divine, thus fulfilling a priestly role, might have formed a professional class of the time. Thorbiorg's story further indicates that local communities also had their own cunning-women offering similar help on a smaller scale using magic and herbs. Martin Carver therefore theorises that it was women such as these that Meaney and Dickinson have found in the ground:

> 'Archaeology, however, opens the door a little wider. It not only shows us a range of the female activists we know must have been present in every society, but even something of their special role – and none was more special than the so-called cunning woman. Don't be misled by the title – this was not a witch or a fortune-teller or the professional magician we know from later centuries. The Anglo-Saxon cunning woman was the equivalent of the female priest, but in an earlier religion and centuries before her first Christian successor.'

The pertinent phrase in Carver's quotation is 'her first Christian successor' as it points to an issue between cunning-women folk-healers and the new religion taking over from paganism. In Thorbiorg's story, we are treated to a dialogue between her and Gudrid which illustrates this issue. Thorbiorg advises Gudrid that it is still possible to help others with healing and ritual whilst remaining a good Christian. Gudrid's view is somewhat different, hinting that the old ways of the cunning-women do not fit within the landscape of Christianity. Gudrid also alludes to the structure of that older path, stating that she learned such things from her step-mother in Iceland. Training to be a healer might thus have been a family tradition with knowledge passing from mother to daughter.

An emerging dissonance between the old and new religions is apparent in Thorbiorg's tale. If Carver is correct and women such as Thorbiorg and her local associates like Gudrid and her step-mother really did form a priestly class, then the Church's attitude towards them becomes clearer. If we look forward, momentarily, to the Middle Ages where priests were exclusively men and healthcare had predominantly moved into masculine hands then we can retroactively speculate that the dissonance grew in intensity.

During the conversion times which spanned from the sixth to twelfth centuries (and arguably later in Northern Europe), Christianity was moving into a pre-existing social structure where women were revered as physicians and more importantly, priests. For the Roman Church, which viewed women as unable and unworthy to perform such roles, a war was waged to specifically demonise folk-healers and demean their status in the eyes of the local populations. By the time they were done, the Church had successfully reframed the identity of cunning-women from one of healer and spiritual counsellor to an altogether different persona of evil 'witch'.

The mechanism for this powerful and wholly successful re-interpretation of the role of women healers was canon law fuelled by propaganda. A number of documents can be traced from as early as Augustine's *On Christian Teaching Book II* (395 AD), through to the spectacular *Malleus Maleficarum* of the fifteenth century that carefully transform Meaney's cunning-women into witches.

Regino of Prum's *Canon Episcopi* is often held as the tipping point that was to turn the whole Western World into a melting pot of witch hysteria. Within just a couple of centuries of its publication, the role of women in community healthcare would not just be usurped by the monasteries but their very lives would be at stake as attitudes became set in a mould of intolerance. Whether Bald and Hildegard realized the seeds of persecution had indeed been planted we may never know, yet there is a curious contingency between their collection of these remedies and the laws that soon followed which wiped the healers out.

The *Canon Episcopi* contains a detailed list of questions for inquisitors to ask of people thought to be seeking help from cunning-women rather than from the clergy. Also, there are queries to be asked of suspected women themselves. Within the descriptions of the women's activities we find evidence, therefore, of what they were doing and the persistence with which local people turned to them in times of need. One question involves the collection of medicinal herbs: 'Have you collected medicinal herbs with evil incantations?'

'Evil incantations' refers to any type of prayer or invocation that names the old gods in favour of the new. The lingering of pagan beliefs was of great concern to the Church and when faced with a tradition of medicine that had its roots in paganism, a plan to appropriate the remedies and reform them in a Christianised frame is not beyond the realms of possibility. This might have been the intention behind our leechbooks. This theory would make sense of the often awkward and incongruous Christianised aspects of some of the remedies. Religious tension is therefore one of the potential issues that contributed to the demise of cunning-women.

The *Canon* and its companion piece by Burchard of Worms specifically mention gender in relation to the continuation of pagan beliefs. At least seventeen claims are made against women, with just one focused upon men. The language used against women is particularly inflammatory and in the next quotation from the *Canon* we see those who still practice the old ways, or who have returned to doing so are marked out as 'wicked women'. Their wickedness is explained in terms of pagan beliefs:

> 'that some wicked women, who have given themselves back to Satan and been seduced by the illusions and phantasms of demons, believe and profess that, in the hours of night, they ride upon certain beasts with Diana, the goddess of pagans, and an innumerable multitude of women, and in the silence of the night

> traverse great spaces of earth, and obey her commands as of their lady, and are summoned to her service on certain nights.'

Here we can discern the emerging narrative that those who believed in paganism were deceived by demons. Diana is mentioned here. She is a Trinitarian goddess linked with her sisters Hecate and Phoebe and was believed to bring fortune in hunting. Before this, she was linked to earlier Indo-European notions of light. The name Diana can be traced through a number of ancient languages to the word 'daylight'. Yet even experiences of Diana are simply illusions of Satan. One might also infer that any actions such as healings attributed to these cunning-women, therefore, would also be seen as the deceptions of the devil. As the document progresses we find increasing focus upon the apparently aberrant behaviours of women and their deceptions. Any good work and healings achieved by cunning-women for their community was therefore being rebranded as the devil's work.

Among these apparent deceptions are further specifically female skills. For example:

> 'Have you ever consented to the vanities which women practice in their woolen work, in their weaving, who when they begin their weaving hope to be able to bring about that with incantations and with their actions that the threads of the warp and of the woof become so intertwined that unless someone uses counter incantations, he will perish totally?'

Weaving and needlework were considered great skills, comparable in prestige and supernatural power to the continental stone masons. Weaving as a motif of deity existed in the folkloric personifications of the Norns, also known as the Fates. They were personifications of another triple goddess weaving the destiny of mankind; although this does not necessarily imply a determinist cosmology it does hint at an early understanding of divine law and accountability. Two of the sisters, *Urðr* and *Verðandi*, witness the beginning of a person's life and measure its worth and action. *Skuld* is responsible for the manner of its ending according to how that life was lived. This implies a karmic, aetiological element whereby a life is evaluated with any negative debts being paid in the manner of death.

The three Norns are depicted on an Anglo-Saxon artefact called the Franks Casket. In Germany, they are known as the *Matrones*, indicating a possible Goddess or Mother cult associated with these three founding Mothers which stretches back to antiquity. In Roman religion, they were called *Nona, Decima* and *Morta*. *Nona* spun the thread of a life, *Decima* measured the thread and *Morta* cut it.

One story of the Norns visiting a baby is recounted in the legend of the *Norna-Gestr*. Here, a Danish hero was blessed with the arrival of these three priestesses at the time of his birth. A visitation by three powerful individuals at the birth of heroes is a recurrent myth within many religious traditions. In this case, the Norns came to give him gifts and inform his parents of his potential life. It is told that the oldest Norn, *Skuld*, was insulted by the company of guests and cursed the baby by aligning his fate with a candle's flame, so that when the flame went out, his life would end. The other two Norns bound the magic of *Skuld* from doing harm to the child and gave the candle to the mother for safekeeping. Years later, the hero converted to Christianity and the old candle was thought to be nothing more than pagan superstition. Lighting the candle would be a demonstration of the hero's new faith, so he lit the flame. But, so it is told, the magic was intact and *Skuld* cut the thread of his life when the candle waned. These personifications may be evidence of humanity's first attempts at personifying the concept of a divine law.

Evidence that the Fates or Norns continued to be revered by women is found in the *Canon Episcopi* which asks:

> 'Have you done as some women are wont to do at certain times of the year? That is, have you prepared the table in your house and set on the table your food and drink, with three knives, that if those three sisters whom past generations and old-time foolishness called the Fates should come they may take refreshment there,'

We begin to see how the Church was viewing the traditional beliefs of the female healers. The old laws of the Fates and the high regard in which cunning-women were held was being directly challenged by new canon law as evidenced within the *Canon Episcopi*. Yet the questions transcribed within the document are not all to be asked of the women themselves but rather of those who associate with them, respect them, look to them for help and who live by their example. It is the common people who are being addressed within this document. The *Canon Episcopi* was the first document to overtly plant the notion in the minds of communities that certain women, gifted in traditional healing and respected for their weaving and needlework were 'wicked'.

Threads, linens, wool and further items relating to weaving and needlework have been discovered interred with Meaney's cunning-women. In April 2016, a seventh century Anglo-Saxon cemetery was discovered near Stonehenge on Salisbury Plain. Within the fifty-five graves, there was one female inhumation with all the now-familiar hallmarks of a healer, yet including a number of small cylindrical boxes with the remains of thread and fabric inside. It has been suggested that these were the repositories for 'weaving spells'. This theory is currently disputed and there seems little way of establishing its credibility. But as a final example of the wider importance of Bald's *Leechbook III* and *Lacnunga*, I would offer the following two remedies as food for thought:

'Wið ceocadle nim þone hweorfan þe wif mid spinnað, bind on his sweoran mid wyllenan þræde ond swile innan mid hate gate meolce, him biþ sel.'

'For an ailment of the cheek, take the whorl with which women spin, bind it onto his neck with woolen thread, and let him gargle with sheep's milk, he will be better.'

'Wið ðon ðe wif færunga adumbige, genim pollegian ond gnid to duste ond in wulle bewind, allege under þæt wif, hyre bið sona sel.'

> 'For when a woman becomes suddenly dumb, take pennyroyal and crumble it to dust and wind it in wool, lay it under the woman, she will soon be well.'

Both remedies are particularly amuletic. In the first, the whorl used for weaving is bound to the neck with woolen thread to bring about healing. With no pharmacological ingredients, the whorl was likely considered a powerful amulet for healing. In the second cure, pennyroyal wrapped in wool is to be lain below the women suddenly struck mute. Sudden dumbness was viewed as a supernatural occurrence, often the result of a curse and so a protective object to ward off the negative intention may have been considered efficacious. We find many references in spiritual texts to sudden unexplained dumbness being the consequence of negative supernatural intention. In the Bible for example, Gabriel struck Zachariah dumb for his disbelief in the power of God.

I would suggest, however, that the remedy for a woman's sudden dumbness might point to a very early understanding of a particular nervous complaint. Sudden onset of muteness is often a major symptom for what we today term catalepsy. Further symptoms can present as physical rigidity and a trance like state. St Teresa of Avila suffered catalepsy in 1539 due to the stress of being incarcerated in a convent and stress is thought to be the main cause of catalepsy in previously well patients. Also, women are more susceptible:

> 'More particularly is this true of females, in whom some form of menstrual derangement will generally he found to have preceded the cataleptic affection.'
>
> (Hugh Chisholm, *Encyclopaedia Britannica*)

Chisholm then goes on to explain that catalepsy often follows a time of shock, fright or a sustained period of depression. The Old English remedy seems to have taken into account that women suffer this illness more than men, and even more, with the inclusion of pennyroyal, a known emmenagogue used in many 'women's' remedies seems to demonstrate Chisholm's research that catalepsy has a connection with menstruation. But would wrapping pennyroyal in wool and putting it beneath the bed really help?

We are told in the 1835 July issue of the *Boston Medical Journal* that affixing leeches to the temples and labia treated a certain Mrs Finn who suffered from nervous cataleptic symptoms including sudden dumbness. Today it is understood that catalepsy usually diminishes without the need of medical intervention, especially without leaches on the labia. A period of rest is often all that is required.

The woollen amulet placed beneath the women indicates that a time of rest was probably recommended, with the amulet contributing feelings of security and hope for future health. One might also speculate that the cunning-woman, taking care of the one struck dumb, sitting by her bedside, winding the wool, singing charms and providing a reassuring presence and possibly a willing ear, might have been useful too. Therefore, the Old English remedy would have served its patient better than the nineteenth century alternative.

It has been my aim within this book to bring to life the forgotten remedies of the Old English healing texts Bald's *Leechbook III* and *Lacnunga*. The herbal elements of the cures are now being analysed by pharmaceutical experts following the delightful happenchance that afforded students at the University of Nottingham the realisation that a modest remedy for sore eyes actually cures the superbug MRSA.

Yet still these texts are approached with trepidation due to their stranger aspects. Few have known what to do with rituals, amulets, nightwalkers and elves except to label them 'folklore' and file them away as an unwelcome interruption to the more reasonable herbal nature of the remedies. Yet I contend that the folkloric magic and superstition are not the nonsense they might appear.

An article in *The Times* from January 26, 2017 reported that scientists have discovered a causal link between 'psychological distress' and 'physical illness'. The health editor Chris Smyth specifies that in relation to cancer, it is now thought that 'misery' activates certain hormonal responses that elevate the likelihood of contracting the disease. If this is the case, then a health service that does not pay due regard to the psychological aspects of physical illness is perhaps fighting a losing battle.

Sometimes, it is the reassurance of stories and hope in something unseen that lends the greatest tool to the health provider's repertoire. Yet today, our sick lie in hospital beds with staff so overworked that even the basic physical necessities go unobserved. We are so accustomed to looking for a physical and thus pharmaceutical intervention to enable us to continue our fast-paced lives that the fuller emotional and psychological landscape is lost and even when given consideration, is verbalised in terms of stress alone.

The Old English folk-healers, or cunning-women, were addressing through ritual and amuletic prescriptions the landscape of mental health by enabling a structure of belief for the mind to engage with. Magic, elves, rituals and the belief in lucky numbers and days of power and the specific ways to dig herbs were not mere superstition, they are evidence that our ancestors knew that the mind needed tending just as much as the body.

The observations and experimentation that led the Old English folk-healers to discover the anti-convulsive properties of lupin required a sophisticated approach to healthcare. To then frame the physical within a wider notion of the psychological by providing meaningful myths and supernatural encounters was not barbaric sorcery, it was a holistic understanding of the needs of human beings when faced with the worst experiences of illness and mortality.

Appendix 1

The Nine Herbs Charm in Old English from Lacnunga

Gemyne ðu mucgwyrt hwæt þu ameldodest,
hwæt þu renadest æt regenmelde
una þu hattest yldost wyrta.
Ðu miht wið III ond wið xxx,
þu miht wiþ attre ond wið onflyge,
þu miht wiþ þa laþan ðe geond lond færð.
Ond þu wegbrade wyrta modor,
eastan openo, innan mihtigu,
ofer ðe crætu curran, ofer ðe cwene reodan,
ofer ðe bryde bryodedon, ofer þe fearras fnærdon,
eallum þu þon wiðstode ond wiðstunedst,
swa ðu wiðstonde attre and onflyge
ond þæm laðan þe geond lond fereð.
Stune hætte þeos wyrt, heo on stane geweox,
stondeð heo wið attre, stunað heo wærce.
Stiðe heo hatte, wiðstunað heo attre,
wreceð heo wraðan, werpeð ut attor.
+ Þis is seo wyrt seo wiþ wyrm gefeaht,
þeos mæg wið attre, heo mæg wið onflyge,
heo mæg wið ða laþan ðe geond lond fereþ.
Fleoh þu nu attorlaeþ, seo læsse ða maran,
seo mare þa læssan oððæt him beigra bot sy.
Gemyne þu mægðe, hwæt þu ameldodest,
hwæt ðu geændadest æt alorforda;
þæt næfre for gefloge feorh ne gesealde

syþðan him mon mægðan to mete gegyrede.
Þis is seo wyrt ðe wergulu hatte,
ðas onsænde seolh ofer sæs hrygc
ondan attres oþres to bote.
Ðas VIIII onagon wið nygon attrum.
+ Wyrm com snican, toslat he nan,
ða genam woden VIIII wuldortanas,
sloh ða þa næddran þæt heo on VIIII tofleah.
Þær geændade æppel ond attor,
þæt heo næfre ne wolde on hus bugan.
+ Fille ond finule, felamihtigu twa,
þa wyrte gesceop witig drihten,
halig on heofonum, þa he hongode,
sette ond sænde on VII worolde
earmum ond eadigum eallum to bote.
Stondeð heo wið wærce, stunað heo wið attre,
seo mæg wið III ond wið XXX,
wið feondes hond ond wið heabregde,
wið malscrunge minra wihta.
+ Nu magon þas VIIII wyrta wið nygon wuldorgeflogegum,
wið VIIII attrum ond wið nygon onflygnum,
wið ðy readan attre, wið ðy runlan attre,
wið ðy hwitan attre, wið ðy hæwenan attre,
wið ðy geolwan attre, wið ðy grenan attre,
wið ðy wonnan attre, wið ðy wedenan attre,
wið ðy brunan attre, wið ðy basewan attre,
Wið wyrmgeblæd, wið wætergeblæd,
wið þorngeblæd, wið þystelgeblæd,
wið ysgeblæd, wið attorgeblæd,
gif ænig attor eastan fleogan
oððe ænig norðan genægan cume
oððe ænig westan ofer werðeode.
+ Crist stod ofer alde ængan cundes.
Ic ana wat ea rinnende
ond þa nygon nædran nu behealdað;

motan ealle weoda nu wyrtum aspringan,
sæs toslupan, eal sealt wæter,
ðonne ic þis attor of ðe geblawe.
Mucgcwyrt, wegbrade þe eastan open sy, lombes cyrse, attorlaðan, mageðan, netelan, wudusuræppel, fille ond finul, ealde sapan, gewyrc to duste, mængc wiþ þa sapan ond wiþ þæs æpples wor, wyrc slypan of wætere ond of axsan, genim finol, wyl on þære slyppan ond beþe mid ðan gemonge þonne he þa sealfe ondo, ge ær ge æfter. Sing þæt galdor on æcre þara wyrta, III ær he hy wyrce ond on þone æppel eal swa; ond singe þon men in þone muð ond in þa earan buta ond on ða wunde þæt ilce gealdor ær he þa sealfe ondo.

Appendix 2

The Cure for MRSA

(Please do not re-create this charm. The experts at Nottingham University are working on a synthetic, hygienic form.)

> 'Work an eye salve for a wen, take cropleek and garlic, of both equal quantities, pound them well together, take wine and bullocks gall, of both equal quantities, mix with a leek, put this then into a brazen vessel, let it stand nine days in the brass vessel, wring out through a cloth and clear it well, put it into a horn, and about night time apply with a feather to the eye; the best leechdom.'

More information is available from Dr Christina Lee, School of English, on:
Tel: +44 (0)115 846 7194
Email: christina.lee@nottingham.ac.uk

Dr Freya Harrison in the School of Life Sciences
Email: freya.harrison@nottingham.ac.uk

Emma Rayner – Media Relations Manager
Tel: +44 (0)115 951 5793
Email: emma.rayner@nottingham.ac.uk

Bibliography

Adams, Jeffrey. & Williams, Eric., *Mimetic Desire: Essays on Narcissism in German Literature from Romanticism to Postmodernism*, (Studies in German Literature Linguistics, 29 Oct 1995).

Auzias, Dominique. & Labourdette, Jean-Paul., *Best of Bretagne,* (2014 Petit Futé avec photos).

Avens, Roberts., *Imagination is Reality*, (Spring Publications Inc, Putnam, Connecticut, 1980)

Avila, Teresa., *The collected works of St. Teresa of Avila Volume One*, (ICS Publications, Washington, D.C. 1987).

Bates, Brian., *The Real Middle Earth: Magic and Mystery in the Dark Ages,* (Pan Books, 2002).

Bates, Brian., *The Wisdom Of The Wyrd: Teachings for today from our ancient past*, (Rider, 1996).

Burke, Raymond L.; et al., '*Mariology: A Guide for Priests, Deacons, Seminarians, and Consecrated Persons.* (Queenship Publishing/Seat of Wisdom Books, 2008).

Cameron, Michael. L., *Bald's Leechbook and cultural interactions in Anglo-Saxon England,* (Anglo-Saxon England, 1990, pp 5-12).

Cameron, Micheal. L., *Bald's Leechbook: its sources and their use in its compilation,* (Anglo-Saxon England, 1983, 12, pp 153-182).

Campbell, Joseph., *Myths To Live By*, (Souvenir Press Ltd, 1973).

Campbell, Josie, P., *Popular Culture in the Middle Ages*, (University of Wisconsin Press, 1986).

Carver, Dax Donald., *Goddess Dethroned: The Evolution of Morgan le Fay,* (Religious Studies Theses 2006, Paper 1).

Cheetham, Tom., *The World Turned Inside Out: Henry Corbin and Islamic Mysticism,* (Spring Journal Books, Woodstock, Connecticut, 2003).

Clemoes, Peter. & Lapidge, Michael., *Anglo-Saxon England*, Volume 12, (Cambridge University Press, 1986).

BIBLIOGRAPHY

David-Neel, Alexandra., *Initiations and Initiates in Tibet*, (Rider and Company LTD, 1931).

Dickinson, Tania., *An Anglo-Saxon "Cunning Woman" from Bidford-on-Avon,* (cited in The Archaeology of Anglo-Saxon England: Basic Readings, edited by Catherine E. Karkov, 1999).

Falconer, Rachel. & Renevey, Denis. (eds)., *Medieval and Early Modern Literature, Science and medicine*, (Tubingan, 2013).

Grattan, H. & Singer, C., *Anglo-Saxon Magic and Medicine,* (Oxford University Press, 1952).

Greenwood, S., *The Nature of Magic: An Anthropology of Consciousness,* (Berg, Oxford, New York, 2005).

Greenwood, Susan., *The Anthropology of Magic*, (Berg, Oxford, New York, 2009).

Greenwood, Susan., Magic, *Witchcraft And The Otherworld,* (Berg, Oxford, New York, 2000).

Grendon, Felix., *The Anglo-Saxon Charms,* (The Journal of American Folklore Vol. 22, No. 84, Apr. - Jun., 1909).

Hand, Wayland,. *Magical Medicine: The Folkloric Component of Medicine in the Folk Belief,* (University of California Press, 1992).

Henry, Solomon., *Anglo-Saxon leechcraft: An historical sketch of early English Medicine,* (British Medical Association, Wellcome, 1912).

Hillyer, C., *Blood Banking and Transfusion Medicine: Basic Principles & Practice,* (Churchill Livingstone, Second Edition, 2006).

Jolly, K., *Popular Religion in Late Saxon England: Elf Charms in Context,* (University of North Carolina Press, 1996)

Kieckhefer, R., *Magic in the Middle Ages,* (Cambridge University Press, 2000).

Kneller, J., *Kant and the Power of Imagination,* (Cambridge Univeristy Press, 2007).

Kors, A & Peters, E., *Witchcraft in Europe 400-1700,* (University of Pennsylvania Press, Philadelphia, 2001).

Linsell, T., *Anglo-Saxon Mythology, Migration and Magic,* (Anglo-Saxon Books, 1994)..

McCoy, D., *Norse-Mythology.org*

Pettit, E., *Anglo-Saxon remedies, charms and prayers*, (Lewiston, N.Y, Edwin Mellen Press, 2001).

Pollington, S., *Leechcraft, Early English Charms, Plantlore and Healing,* (Anglo-Saxon Books, 2000).

Raff, J., *Jung and the Alchemical Imagination,* (Nicolas-Hays, Inc, Berwick, Maine, 2000).

Reynolds, A., Anglo-Saxon Deviant Burial Customs, (Oxford University Press, First Edition, 2014).

Richardson, H., *Slug on a thorn*, (*Pitt Rivers Museum Website,* 2013).

Rodriguez de la Sierra, L., *Origin of the myth of vampirism*, (Journal of the Royal Society of medicine, 1998).

Sayer, D. & Dickinson, S., *Reconsidering obstetric death and female fertility in Anglo-Saxon England*, (World Archaeology, 2013).

Sinclair Rohde, E., *The Old English herbals*, (Createspace Publishing, 2010).

Sircus, M., *Transdermal-Magnesium*, (Phaelos Books & Mediawerks; First Edition, 2007).

Spencer, R. L., *The Craft of the Warrior*, (Frog Ltd, Berkeley California, Second Edition, 2005).

Voss, A., *Magic, Astrology and Music: The background to Marsillio Ficino's astrological music therapy and his role as a renaissance magus,* (unpublished work, 1992).

Wright, T., *The Worship of The Generative Powers: During the Middle Ages of Western Europe*, (Createspace, 2011).

Yelyr, R., *The Whip And The Rod - An Account Of Corporal Punishment Among All Nations*, (Candler Press, 2013).

Index

INDEX